DIET AND HEART DISEASE

DIET AND HEART DISEASE
A round table of factors

Second edition

Edited by Dr Margaret Ashwell OBE

Published by Chapman & Hall
for the British Nutrition Foundation

CHAPMAN & HALL
London . Weinheim . New York . Tokyo . Melbourne . Madras

Published by Chapman & Hall, 2–6 Boundary Row, London SE1 8HN, UK

Chapman & Hall, 2–6 Boundary Row, London SE1 8HN, UK

Chapman & Hall GmbH, Pappelallee 3, 69469 Weinheim, Germany

Chapman & Hall USA, 115 Fifth Avenue, New York, NY 10003, USA

Chapman & Hall Japan, ITP-Japan, Kyowa Building, 3F, 2-2-1 Hirakawacho, Chiyoda-ku, Tokyo 102, Japan

Chapman & Hall Australia, 102 Dodds Street, South Melbourne, Victoria 3205, Australia

Chapman & Hall India, R. Seshadri, 32 Second Main Road, CIT East, Madras 600 035, India

First edition 1993
Published by:
The British Nutrition Foundation
52–54 High Holborn House
High Holborn
London WC1V 6RQ
Second edition 1997

Typeset in 10/12pt Helvetica by Columns Design Ltd, Reading

ISBN-13: 978-94-010-6527-6 e-ISBN-13: 978-94-009-0087-5
DOI: 10.1007/978-94-009-0087-5

A catalogue record for this book is available from the British Library

Library of Congress Catalog Card Number: 96–86099

∞ Printed on permanent acid-free text paper, manufactured in accordance with ANSI/NISO Z39.48-1992 (Permanence of Paper)

CONTENTS

The Round Table Model colour plate section appears between pages 16 and 17

ACKNOWLEDGEMENTS

The Round Table Model was devised by Anne Halliday (now Mrs Anne de la Hunty) and Dr Margaret Ashwell. This book was originally based on the series of four Briefing Papers produced by the British Nutrition Foundation during 1992 and 1993. Expert help for these was provided by Dr Peter Elwood, Professor David Galton, Professor Colin Berry and Professor Mike Gurr. The Foundation's Scientific Advisory Committee was responsible for developing the four Papers.

The first edition of this book was written by Dr Margaret Ashwell, Anne Halliday, Dr Michèle Sadler and Ursula Arens. The second edition of this book has been fully updated and edited by Dr Margaret Ashwell OBE.

ABBREVIATIONS USED IN THE TEXT

apoA	apoprotein A
apoB	apoprotein B
BMI	body mass index
BP	blood pressure
CETP	cholesterol ester transfer protein
CHD	coronary heart disease
CM	chylomicron
CM-R	chylomicron remnant
CRG	Coronary Review Group of the Committee on Medical Aspects of Food Policy (UK)
CVD	cardiovascular disease
DNA	deoxyribonucleic acid
DHA	docosahexaenoic acid
DRV	dietary reference value(s)
EDRF	endothelium-derived relaxing factor
EFA	essential fatty acids
EPA	eicosapentaenoic acid
GI	glycaemic index
Hcy	plasma homocysteine
HDL	high density lipoprotein
kcal	kilocalories
kJ	kilojoules
Lp(a)	lipoprotein(a)
LDL	low density lipoprotein
LDL/HDL	low density lipoprotein/high density lipoprotein ratio
LPL	lipoprotein lipase(s)
MRFIT	multiple risk factor intervention trial
MUFA	monounsaturated fatty acid(s)
NO	nitric oxide
NSP	non-starch polysaccharides
PUFA	polyunsaturated fatty acid(s)
RCT	randomized controlled trial
RS	resistant starch
SFA	saturated fatty acid(s)
SMR	standardized mortality rates
TG	triglycerides
VLDL	very low density lipoproteins
WHR	waist to hip circumference ratio
WHTR	waist circumference to height ratio

INTRODUCTION

There is no doubt that coronary heart disease (CHD) is a multifactorial disorder. Family history, race, sex and age all play a part but can be considered as uncontrollable factors. Among the controllable factors, due attention must be given to smoking, exercise, stress and, of course, diet.

This book focuses on diet and CHD, not necessarily because it is the most important factor, but because it is the one component which can be modified by all. Hence the enormous attention devoted to it by the health professionals, the media and the Food Industry.

A major problem is that there is considerable confusion about individual dietary components and the role they play in CHD (British Nutrition Foundation, 1992a,b,c; 1993). The simple message that fats are 'bad' and fibre is 'good' has undergone much refinement in recent years and the public cannot be expected to understand that while certain fatty acids have a protective effect, others do not, and that the interactions between other dietary components such as antioxidants and prooxidants can determine the balanced effect.

We set out to develop a model that could help to explain several important basic concepts about CHD and which could then be used to explain the role of different dietary components. An important element of our approach was that it had to be scientifically accurate while being simple to interpret.

We therefore decided that the pathological events of CHD could be divided into three main sections – arterial injury, fibrous plaque formation and thrombus formation with subsequent heart attack. The main physiological risk conditions such as blood pressure and cholesterol and fibrinogen levels were then allocated to the particular pathological event they are thought to influence. In some cases there was more than one.

We considered the dietary factors individually and assigned them to a particular disease event/physiological condition/dietary component triad. In several cases, a dietary component was allocated to more than one triad.

Thus, we built up the complete Round Table Model that is shown in the colour section. We believe that this model illustrates the following points about diet and CHD:

- There are several pathological stages each influenced by different physiological conditions and different dietary components.
- No one dietary component acts in isolation from other components and, in many cases, a physiological risk factor will be influenced by a balance of several dietary components.
- Several dietary components can influence several different physiological conditions, not necessarily by the same mechanisms.

Above all, the Round Table Model emphasizes over and over again the original philosophy of King Arthur when he placed his knights at a round table to show that no one knight took precedence over another. In terms of their relationships to heart disease, it is the integrated role of the whole diet which is important and we hope that the Round Table Model will help to strengthen this concept.

Introduction to the second edition

In the 3 years since the first edition of this book was published, the Round Table Model has received wide acclaim. The model has been described as a teaching tool which helps the reader to grasp an extremely complex subject and a concise and practical means of simplifying the multiple and complex factors associated with CHD.

I have been amazed at how much new evidence has been published in this short period of time on the relationship between diet and CHD. In this respect, the Round Table Model has helped me to assess each piece of evidence in the context of the model and to work out how it influences the interrelationships portrayed in the Round Table Model. I am very grateful then to have this opportunity to edit the second edition of this book so that subtle, but important, changes can be made which reflect the new scientific evidence and the new Reports which have been published in the past 3 years.

Dr Margaret Ashwell OBE, 1996

SUMMARY

1. Coronary Heart Disease (CHD) is a major cause of death, particularly in the Western World, but increasingly so elsewhere. There are wide variations in death rates due to CHD around the world; those in the UK are among the highest. CHD is predominantly a disease of old age. The peak age of deaths from CHD is 70 to 74 years in men and 75 to 79 years in women.

2. The development of CHD can be viewed simplistically as a three-stage process.

   The initial arterial injury is followed by deposition of lipid and cell material (atherosclerosis) and small blood clots (thrombi) which contribute to the build-up of fibrous plaque. Instability in the plaque triggers the formation of a major blood clot (thrombus) in the already narrowed artery. This gives the potential for the blood and oxygen supply to the heart muscle to be blocked completely which will result in myocardial infarction (heart attack).

3. Prospective trials have shown that people with high blood pressure, high levels of low density lipoprotein cholesterol, low levels of high density lipoprotein cholesterol, high levels of plasma fibrinogen and high levels of plasma insulin carry an increased risk of subsequently developing CHD. Low levels of some plasma antioxidants have been shown in cross-sectional studies to be associated with higher CHD mortality rates.

4. Each of the three stages of heart disease can be influenced by several physiological conditions (e.g. high blood pressure, high plasma levels of lipids and low plasma levels of antioxidants). It is these conditions with which the controllable (or behavioural) factors, including dietary factors, can interact.

5. The uncontrollable (or background) factors for CHD are family history, maleness, increasing age, racial origin and, possibly, factors occurring in early life such as birthweight and growth in the first year of life which cannot be modified once achieved.

6. The abnormal physiological conditions which affect the frequency and severity of injury to the coronary arteries include increased blood pressure, increased lipid oxidation, an increased tendency for platelet aggregation and an increased inflammatory response. Blood pressure is increased by high salt intakes, the ratio of sodium to potassium intake, increased alcohol intake and obesity. Lipid oxidation is affected by the oxidizability of the fatty acids in the low density lipoprotein particle and the balance between pro-oxidants and antioxidants. Increased platelet aggregation and increased inflammation are further factors which increase the likelihood of arterial injury.

7. The build-up of fibrous plaque on the inside of the injured arterial wall is determined by abnormal physiological conditions which affect both lipid and thrombus deposition in the plaque, i.e. an increased atherogenic lipid profile, increased plasma fibrinogen and other factors influencing the blood clotting pathway and possibly increased plasma insulin levels. Plasma cholesterol in atherogenic lipoproteins can be reduced by decreasing certain dietary saturated fatty acids, substituting monounsaturated fatty acids or n-6 polyunsaturated fatty acids for certain saturated fatty acids or by increasing the amount of alcohol and soluble non-starch polysaccharides (fibre) in the diet. Plasma fibrinogen levels do not appear to be particularly influenced by diet, although a moderately increased alcohol intake is associated with lower levels of plasma fibrinogen in cross-sectional studies. Resistance to the action of insulin and the consequently increased plasma levels of insulin is a condition associated with 'central' deposition of fat. This can be reversed by exercise and weight loss. Smaller, more frequent meals may also help to reduce average plasma insulin levels. Plasma homocysteine levels appear to influence fibrous plaque formation and increased intakes of folate and folic acid can be beneficial.

8. The formation of a major thrombus and the severity of a heart attack is influenced by factors affecting blood coagulation and regularity of the heartbeat. Fish oils and moderate alcohol intake can reduce the tendency for blood to coagulate through their effects on platelet aggregation. Some evidence suggests that saturated fatty acids may increase the tendency towards irregular heart beat in men with heart disease and that fish oils may have opposite effect.

9. The effect of diet on the risk of CHD will be due to the integrated effect of all dietary factors, whether they individually promote or protect against CHD. CHD cannot therefore be attributed to any single component of the diet. The Round Table Model for Diet and CHD acknowledges this important fact. It provides a model which shows where and how the individual dietary components might act and also demonstrates the importance of interactions which might take place.

10. Dietary advice for the general population should include advice to eat more fruit and vegetables including pulses and legumes, more starchy foods such as potatoes, rice, bread and pasta, and more oil-rich fish. For men aged over 40 years and postmenopausal women, low intakes of alcohol should be advocated in regular amounts. There should be advice to eat more reduced-fat rather than full-fat dairy products, more reduced fat rather than full-fat meat products and to use less salt. The most important dietary advice that can be given, however, is that food should be enjoyed and that maximum enjoyment can be achieved by taking an interest in food and exploring the wide variety of food and drink that is available today.

1

EPIDEMIOLOGY

Coronary heart disease (CHD) is a major cause of death in Western countries, and increasingly so in Eastern European and some developing countries. There are wide variations in death rates due to CHD around the world; those in the United Kingdom (UK) are among the highest.

CHD is predominantly a disease of old age. The peak age of death from CHD is 70–74 years in men and 75–79 years in women. However, CHD is a major cause of premature death (before 65 years) in men.

The term CHD covers angina pectoris (severe chest pain on exertion or excitement), acute myocardial infarction (heart attack) and sudden death. The underlying condition, atherosclerosis, causes obstruction in the arteries supplying the heart, resulting in reduced blood flow to the heart muscle.

Angina is caused by inadequate blood flow. If the blood flow is blocked completely by formation of a thrombus (blood clot) in an already narrowed artery, a heart attack occurs. Death occurs within a few hours in about half those suffering a heart attack.

CHD is a major form of cardiovascular disease (CVD), a term which also includes stroke and peripheral atherosclerosis.

1.1 WORLDWIDE COMPARISONS

1.1.1 All-age mortality

Some of the variations in death rates from CHD may arise due to different criteria for classifying causes of death between countries. Though the UK has a high death rate from CHD, life expectancy is among the highest in the world.

Figure 1.1 shows standardized mortality rates (SMR) (deaths/100 000 population) from all causes and from CHD for men. The rates have been standardized to a world population to allow comparison between countries with different distributions of age groups within the population. This shows that death rates from all causes and from CHD were, at the time, highest in the Union of Soviet Socialist Republics (USSR).

Death rates in Scotland and Northern Ireland are also high and this is reflected in the life expectancies from age 15 (which excludes the effects of high infant mortality rates) for these countries (Figure 1.2).

Although men in England and Wales have a greater chance of dying from CHD than men in the United States of America (USA), they can expect to

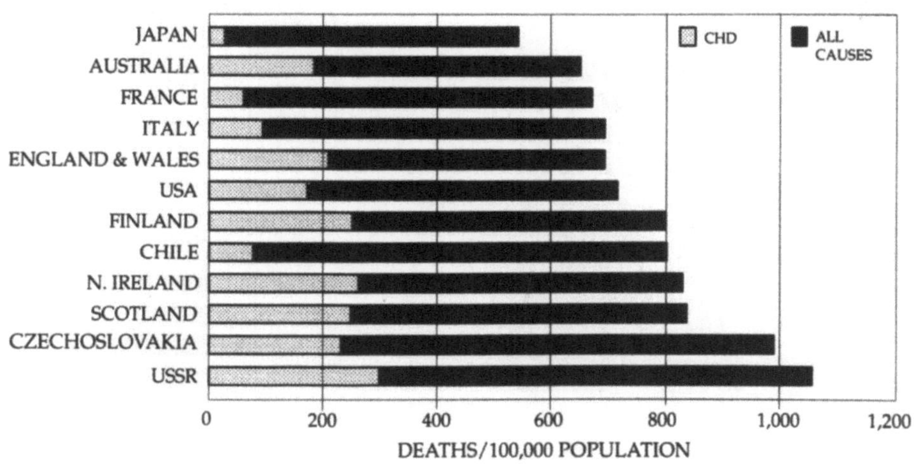

Figure 1.1 Standardized mortality rates from CHD and from all causes (men) in selected countries, 1986–1988. (Source: World Health Organization, 1989.)

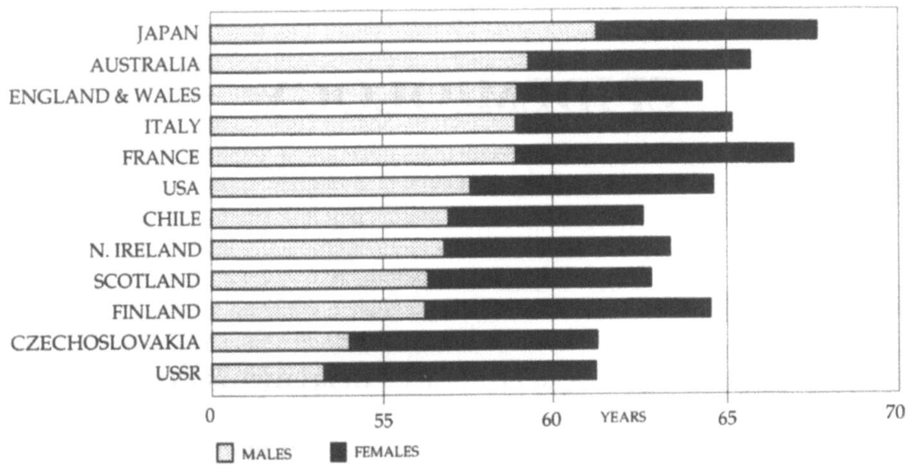

Figure 1.2 Life expectancy from 15 years in selected countries, 1986–1988. (Source World Health Organization, 1989.)

live longer before they suffer a fatal heart attack. Men in Japan have a low average death rate and a very low death rate from CHD (Figure 1.1) which is reflected in their greater life expectancy (Figure 1.2).

Women tend to live longer than men (Figure 1.2) and have lower standardized mortality rates (Figure 1.3). A smaller proportion of women die from CHD, but a cross-country comparison shows a rank order fairly similar to that for men.

1.1.2 Premature mortality

Though death rates from CHD rise rapidly in older men and women, CHD is a major cause of premature death in men. When CHD mortality rates in men and women aged 30–69 years are compared (Figure 1.4), Scotland and Northern Ireland hold unenviable positions near the top of the 'league table'.

Premature deaths account for about 26% of all deaths in men and 16% of all deaths in women in the UK. In 1988 in the UK 8% of men and 2% of women who died, died prematurely from CHD.

This can obviously cause much hardship and difficulty for family and dependants.

CHD also causes much illness, since those who survive a heart attack (about half) may experience difficulty and pain during the rest of their lives and are at greater risk of a second heart attack.

1.1.3 Trends with time

Death rates from CHD have been declining in many parts of the world over the past 20 years. However, they have begun to rise in Eastern Europe (Gintner *et al.*, 1995) and in some developing countries.

Countries such as the USA, Australia, Israel, Canada, Japan and New Zealand have seen large falls in premature CHD mortality rates since 1970 (Figure 1.5). Other Western European countries, such as Finland, Norway, Italy and the UK have had smaller reductions over the same period.

In contrast, there have been striking increases

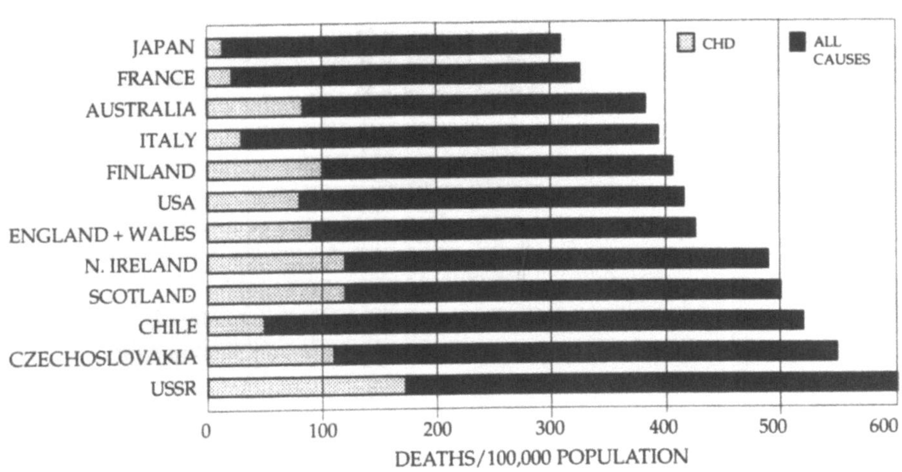

Figure 1.3 Standardized mortality rates from CHD and from all causes (women) in selected countries, 1986–1988. (Source: World Health Organization, 1989.)

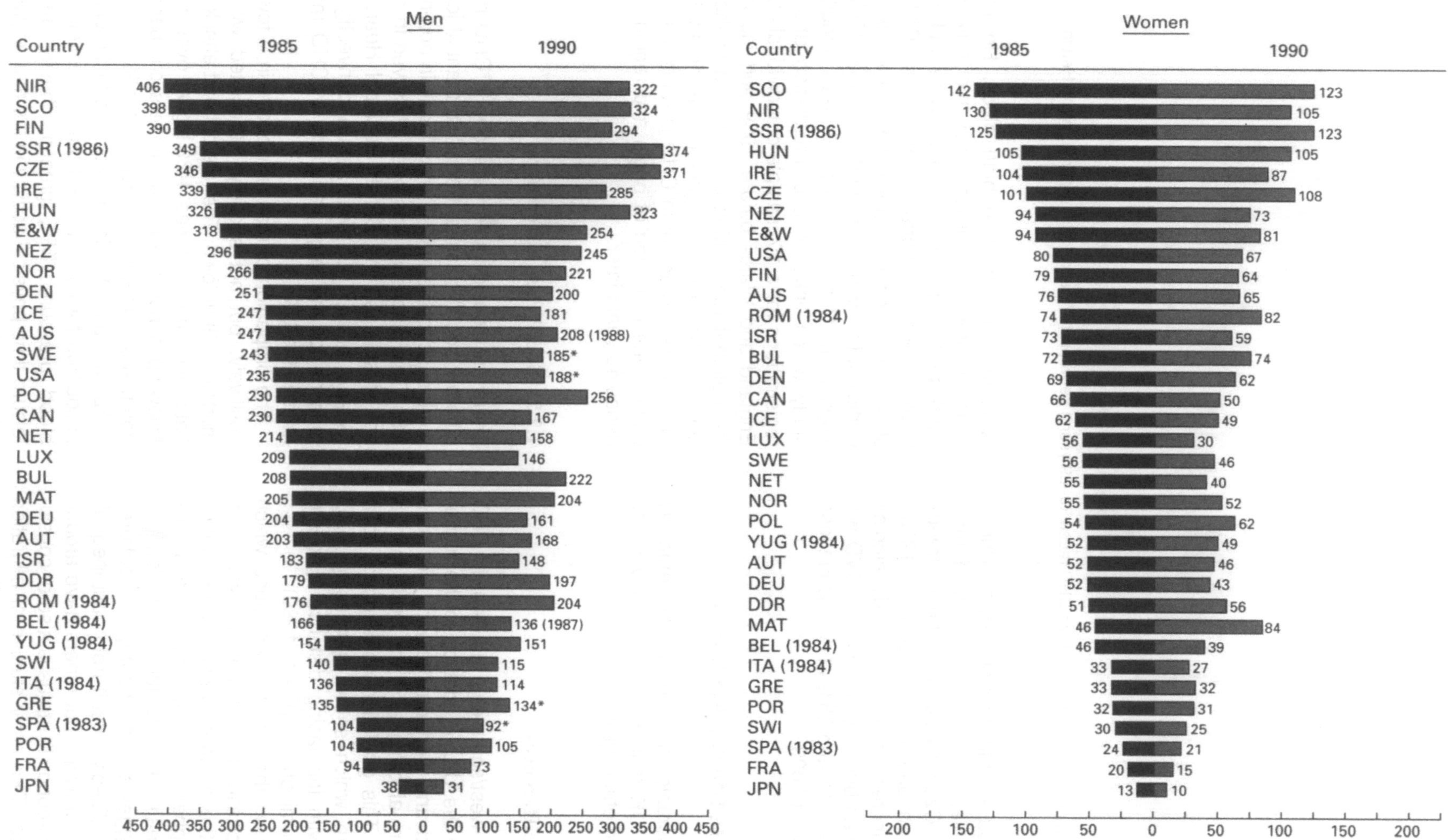

Figure 1.4 Age-standardized mortality from ischaemic heart disease in men and women, 1985 and 1990. Rates are expressed per 100 000 population, aged 30–69 years. * indicates 1989 values. (Source: World Health Organization, 1989; World Health Statistics Annual 1992.)

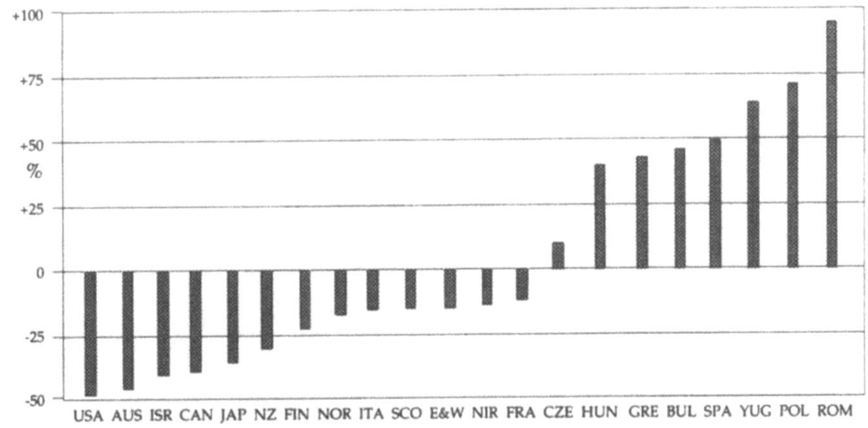

Figure 1.5 Change in male death rates (%) from CHD (aged 30–69 years) between 1970 and 1985. (Source: World Health Organization, 1989.)

during this period in the former Soviet Union, Bulgaria, Romania, Hungary, Poland, former Yugoslavia and Czechoslovakia. These trends exist for both men and women (Gintner, 1995). There are also increases in CVD in developing countries and it has been estimated that CVD will account for between 15 and 25% of deaths in these countries by the year 2000.

1.2 WITHIN THE UNITED KINGDOM

There are considerable variations in CHD mortality rates in different UK regions, and within different social classes and ethnic groups.

1.2.1 Regional differences

There is a north-west/south-east gradient in CHD mortality rates in the UK. In addition to the higher rates in Scotland and Northern Ireland, the rates within England are also higher in the North than in the South East. This gradation corresponds to a worldwide pattern which shows increasing CHD mortality rates with increasing distance from the equator in both hemispheres (Fleck, 1989).

Figure 1.6 shows the regional variations which exist for CHD mortality rates in men and women in the UK. Within these large areas, urban centres tend to have higher rates than rural areas (see Department of Health, 1994 for further details).

It has been suggested that geographical patterns of cardiovascular disease result from past inequalities in standards of living, but others have argued that current socioeconomic status is also of considerable importance. Two early studies of migration within Britain have shown conflicting results. In the British Regional Heart Study (Shaper *et al.*, 1981), the incidence of ischaemic heart disease (IHD) in middle-aged men was more closely related to place of examination than to birth place. However, a national study of proportional mortality during 1969–1972 suggested that birth place had a significant effect on mortality rates from CHD and stroke. In a recent study (Strachan *et al.*, 1995) participants were obtained via the Office of Population Censuses and Surveys longitudinal study which links census information and death registrations for a 1% sample of individuals born in England and Wales before 1939 and included in the national registration in 1939 and in the 1971 census. The results suggested that the south-east to north-west gradient in CHD is related in almost equal parts to region of origin and region of residence 40 years later.

1.2.2 Social class differences

There are considerable variations in CHD rates in different social classes. People in manual jobs are more susceptible to CHD than those in non-manual jobs. This difference has been observed in a number of studies. The British Regional Heart Study (Shaper *et al.*, 1981) was set up to investigate the reasons for the large variations in CHD mortality rates in the UK.

The proportion of manual workers in a town was positively, but not strongly, associated with CHD mortality in that town. The rate of heart attack events (fatal and non-fatal) was 44% higher over a 6-year follow-up period in manual workers compared with non-manual workers (Pocock *et al.*, 1987).

About half of this excess mortality could be accounted for by increased smoking levels, higher blood pressure (BP), greater obesity and less leisure-time physical activity in the manual workers. Interestingly, plasma cholesterol levels were lower in the manual workers than in the non-manual workers (see Chapter 3).

Other studies have also reported higher CHD

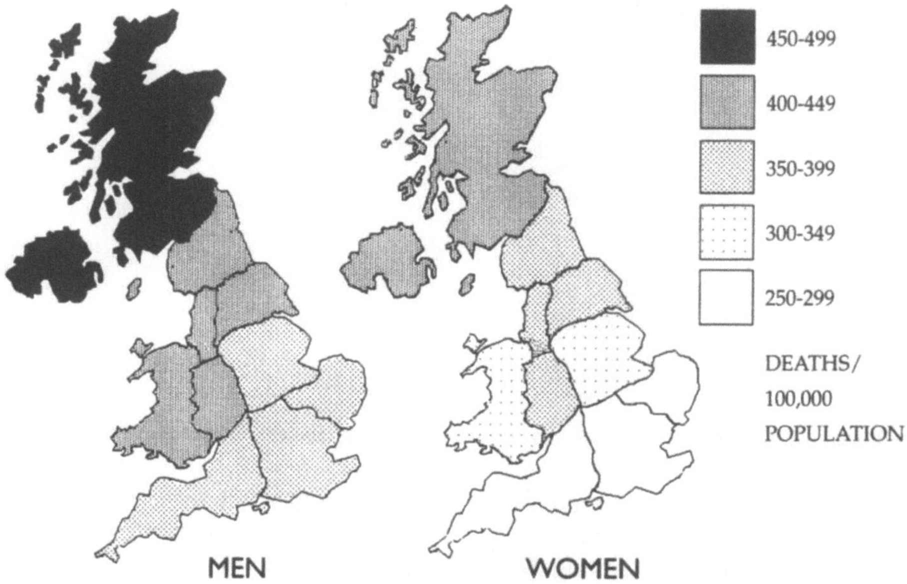

Figure 1.6 Deaths from CHD by UK geographical region in 1987. (Source: Office of Population Censuses and Surveys.)

mortality rates in manual workers. The Whitehall Study of Civil Servants found that the lowest-grade men had three times the mortality of men in the highest grades over the 10-year follow-up period (Marmot *et al.*, 1978).

Men within grades may be a more homogeneous group than the rather diverse social class groupings: this could explain the greater difference observed in this study compared with that in the British Regional Heart Study.

The Whitehall Study of Civil Servants also found higher rates of smoking, more obesity, higher BP and less leisure-time physical activity in the lower grades than in the higher grades, although these factors did not completely explain the differences in mortality between the groups.

Figure 1.7 shows the variations in CHD mortality by social class and sex. There is a consistent trend to increasing mortality, rising from lower than expected in social class I (professional occupations) and social class II (intermediate occupations), through average mortality in social class IIIN (skilled non-manual occupations) to higher than expected in social classes IIIM (skilled manual occupations), social class IV (partly skilled occupations) and social class V (unskilled occupations). The social class differences are slightly more pronounced in women (Department of Health, 1994).

1.2.3 Ethnic group differences

Gujaratis, Punjabis, Bangladeshis and Southern Indians in London have 40% higher CHD mortality rates than UK national averages (McKeigue *et al.*, 1991). Similar findings have been found in a number of different countries around the world (e.g. Singapore, South Africa, Uganda and Fiji).

Figure 1.8 shows the variations in CHD mortality in England and Wales by ethnic origin as assessed

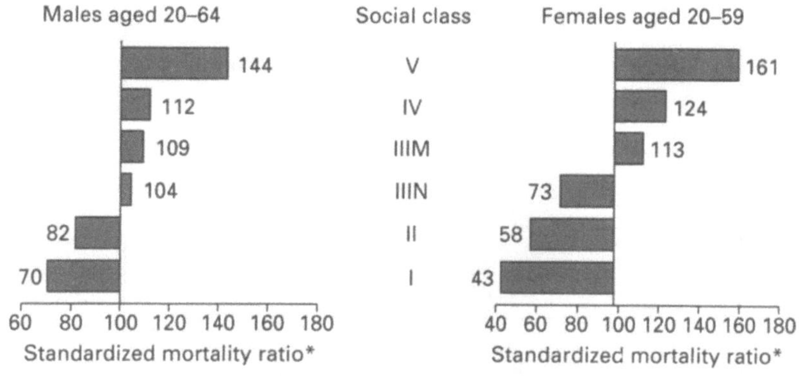

Figure 1.7 Variations in mortality from CHD by social class and sex, Great Britain, 1979–1983. *All values of standardized mortality ratios are significant at the 1% level. (Source: Department of Health, 1994, © Crown Copyright.)

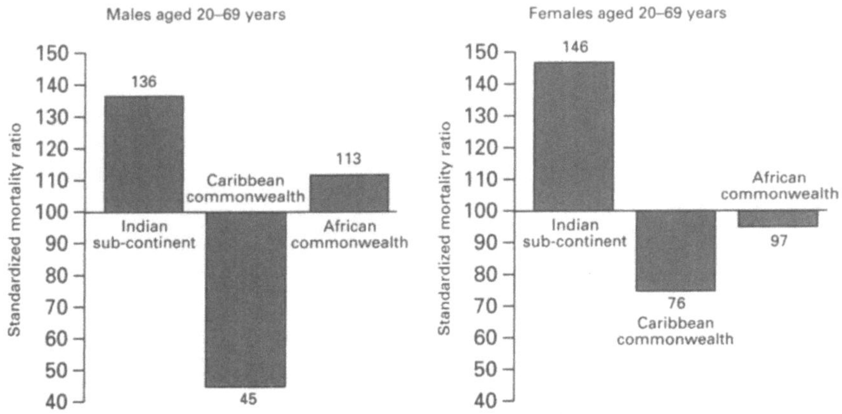

Figure 1.8 Variations in deaths from CHD by sex and ethnic origin, 1979–1983. (Source: Department of Health, 1994, © Crown Copyright.)

by country of birth. Mortality from CHD in men and women aged 20 to 69 born in the Indian sub-continent is 36% and 46% higher than among the population as a whole. In contrast, men and women born in the Caribbean commonwealth have CHD mortality rates which are lower than the general population (Department of Health, 1994), even though their chances of dying from stroke are higher than average.

1.2.4 Trends with time in the UK

The overall reduction in premature mortality in the UK during the past 25 years obscures much larger falls in specific age groups. Figure 1.9 shows the changes in male death rates from CHD for different age groups in England and Wales since 1980. Although absolute death rates in the youngest group are much lower than in older men, the percentage decline in this group has been twice that of the oldest group. The fall in death rates for women has not shown such a marked effect of age. The CHD death rates for Scotland and Northern Ireland have remained consistently higher than those for England and Wales but the declines in death rates have shown broadly similar patterns (Department of Health, 1994).

1.3 CONSIDERATION OF METHODOLOGY

1.3.1 Sources of data

Finding explanations for these observed differences in the distribution of CHD among different groups of people could help to unravel the causes of CHD.

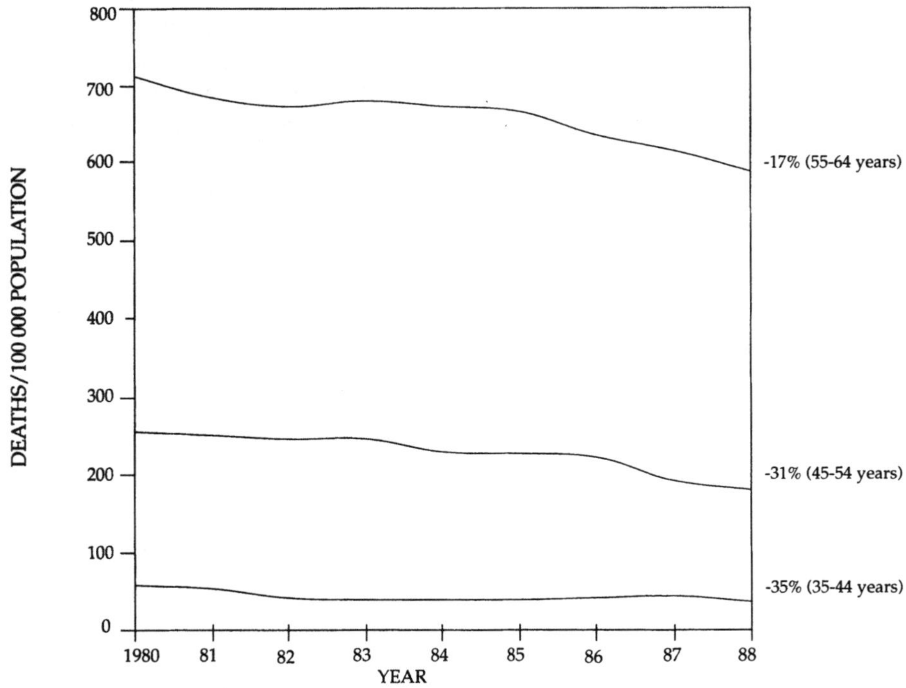

Figure 1.9 Trends in age-specific CGD mortality in men in England and Wales. (Source: Office of Population Censuses and Surveys.)

It is appropriate to focus on studies of human populations. Although a few long-lived animals appear to get atherosclerosis, there seems to be no animal model for heart attack. While animals may provide a basis for studies of metabolic pathways and biological mechanisms, such work cannot constitute a basis for evaluation of mechanisms in human subjects, nor their relevance in disease in communities. Various strategies can be adopted:

(a) Cross-community comparisons

There are large differences in disease rates in different communities and some of these are particularly large between countries. Relating disease rates to differences in dietary intakes is useful and a number of interesting hypotheses have arisen in this way. There are difficulties, however, as the dietary data from different communities may not be truly representative and the disease data may not be directly comparable.

Far more important is the virtual impossibility of linking differences in disease incidence solely to dietary differences. Genetic, behavioural and environmental factors will almost certainly differ and may well be far more important than dietary differences.

(b) Examining trends with time

There have been great changes in mortality from CHD in most countries during the past century. While angina was probably common at the beginning of the century, heart attack seems to have been rare and unrecognized.

It is tempting to look for dietary changes which parallel these changes in disease incidence. Difficulties arise because information on past disease is uncertain and knowledge of past dietary intakes is poor. Even if reliable data were available, the two could not be linked with any degree of certainty because many other relevant factors are likely to have changed concurrently.

Diet is only one aspect of lifestyle and it cannot be considered in isolation. As with comparisons between communities, historical evidence can only draw attention to factors of possible importance which should be investigated by more accurate methods.

(c) Case-control studies

The identification of patients with evidence of a disease and comparison with disease-free subjects is one of the most simple research strategies. It has a limited place in nutritional research because it requires assessment of dietary intakes before onset of the disease. It may be difficult for a patient to remember this clearly in relation to dietary changes which have been made since symptoms of the disease commenced.

The case-control approach has little place in cardiovascular research because around half the subjects who suffer a heart attack die within a few hours. Only a sub-sample of cases survive to be included in a case-control study and these are certainly not representative of all patients with the condition.

(d) Prospective studies

The prospective, cohort, or longitudinal study is the classic tool of the epidemiologist. Baseline measurements of possible associated factors are made and related to subsequent disease events.

The strategy has substantial advantages over other research approaches provided the cohort is sufficiently large and is representative of a defined population and provided the follow up is long-term. The main advantage is that suspected causes can be measured before the disease becomes evident and can be distinguished from effects of the disease.

Whether or not factors show greater-than-chance associations is not the final answer from such studies. The degree to which the predictive power of a factor associated with the disease is independent of other factors must be examined.

In practice it is found that a number of factors are inter-related. Unscrambling these relationships presents great difficulties especially when there are variations in the degree of precision with which each is estimated.

(e) Intervention trials

The Randomized Controlled Trial (RCT) is a powerful tool in medical research. Guidelines for this strategy are well established and if a study is to yield reliable evidence there can be no compromise on the cardinal rules for an RCT, namely:

- random allocation to intervention or control group
- blind assessment of end-points
- complete follow up of subjects.

Unfortunately, it is rarely possible in dietary RCTs to comply with a further important requirement, namely:

- blindness of the participants as to whether they are receiving the intervention measure.

This is achieved in drug trials by the use of a placebo tablet, but in dietary studies use of a dummy foodstuff is impossible.

There are two kinds of intervention trial. Small, short-term studies examine a mechanism or test the association between a dietary factor such as salt intake and a factor known to be predictive of disease, such as altered BP. The more important trials are those which test the relevance of a factor to the incidence of a disease.

While RCTs give strong evidence they also have limitations, particularly in full-scale trials which test a dietary factor against CVD incidence.

A major limitation of dietary RCTs is the difficulty in persuading subjects to make significant change to their dietary intake and maintain this for a sufficient time, while avoiding 'contamination' of the control group. Changes in the two groups must be carefully monitored. It is important to avoid as far as possible changes in factors other than the ones of interest. All the changes which do occur must be monitored.

Secondary prevention trials, based on patients who have already had a cardiovascular event, have some advantages over primary intervention trials, particularly because they require fewer subjects. There are some uncertainties in such trials, in particular whether the disease has advanced too far for a preventive measure to be effective. This may not always be the case and secondary prevention is within the resources of many research groups, while primary prevention is not.

1.3.2 Interpretation of data

A clear distinction must be made between testing a hypothesis defined before a study was set up, and the generation of new hypotheses from data collected for another purpose. The latter is often dismissed under the name 'fishing' or 'dredging' and any associations detected should be tested in further studies.

Firm conclusions should only be based on evidence drawn from several studies. The play of chance can never be ruled out, whatever the level of statistical significance. Consistency in a number of studies is often a better indication of an effect than the results of a single study.

Hence the importance of 'overviews' of studies or 'meta-analyses' of data from a number of different studies. This approach is most appropriate with RCTs, but it is important that data from every relevant RCT is included. Publication bias (papers which report an effect are generally more likely to be accepted by a journal than those which show no effect) makes a neutral overview difficult (Ravnskov, 1992).

One should also look for consistency in the results of studies with different approaches. Confidence is enhanced if prospective studies demonstrate an association between a food item and a disease, if RCTs show a change in the disease incidence in the intervention group, and if these effects are consistent with the results of metabolic studies.

There are difficulties in interpreting the reduction of non-fatal CHD events which are observed in most of the RCTs with dietary fat reduction. No trial has attempted to collect data on all morbid events and the increase in non-CHD deaths makes the interpretation of data on non-fatal CHD events uncertain.

Long-term effects of changing disease incidence would mean that a significant reduction or delay in one disease, such as CHD, would be likely to result in an increase in the incidence of all other diseases at a particular age.

Because of these uncertainties the most reasonable way forward is to base conclusions relating to clinical practice and population control programmes on data relating to survival in trials in CVD. This group of diseases account for the majority of deaths in Western communities and therefore if a dietary or other measure affects the disease it should improve overall survival.

1.4 RISK FACTORS FOR CORONARY HEART DISEASE

1.4.1 Definitions

The purpose of the various types of study described above is to identify factors that are associated with the onset and progression of CHD.

A risk factor is able to predict, to some extent, the CHD mortality rate in a prospective trial, excluding the possibility that it may be a consequence of the disease. Associated factors identified by cross-sectional trials or retrospective studies are not strictly risk factors as they have not been shown to precede the onset of the disease.

Having identified risk factors, intervention trials attempt to modify the risk of the disease by modifying the risk factor. If both the risk of the disease and the risk of death from all causes are reduced, the factor is assumed to be a causal factor in the development of the disease but this assumption is not always valid.

Prevention of the disease should be targeted at risk and causal factors which have been shown to contribute to the onset and development of the disease and are not merely a side effect of the disease themselves.

The risk of CHD cannot be predicted from a single risk factor.

CHD is a multifactorial disease which arises out of interaction of different combinations of risk factors. Particular combinations can be especially atherogenic and these interactions may explain some of the observed anomalies in cross-cultural comparisons. Within individuals the potency of different factors will be modulated to some degree by individual susceptibility (see Chapter 4).

1.4.2 Categorization and interactions

Risk factors can be categorized as:

- physiological factors (second ring in the Round Table Model in the colour section)
- uncontrollable (or background) factors (third ring in the Round Table Model in the colour section)
- controllable (or behavioural) factors.

Figure 1.10 summarizes the relationships and interactions between behavioural and physiological factors.

Many of the behavioural factors exert their effects through a number of different physiological risk factors. For example obesity, defined as having a body mass index (BMI) greater than 30, particularly with excess central fat deposition, can lead to high BP, increased plasma insulin levels and increased plasma cholesterol levels – all physiological factors that increase the risk of CHD. Sometimes a behavioural factor can have a beneficial effect on some risk factors, yet it can increase risk in other areas. Alcohol is a good example. Heavy, irregular alcohol drinking ('binge' drinking) can increase blood pressure, but regular consumption of moderate alcohol can reduce the build-up of fibrous plaque and reduce likelihood of a blood clot.

1.4.3 Putting the benefits of modifying risk factors into perspective

With such a multi-factorial disease as CHD, it is not surprising that there have been so few attempts to summarize the benefits of modifying the different controllable risk factors.

Manson *et al.* (1992) made an attempt at doing this on the basis of either meta-analyses or reviews of the larger and more rigorous studies. They concluded that giving up smoking, cholesterol reduction, control of high blood pressure, maintenance of ideal body weight, and regular exercise all appeared to reduce the risk of a first heart attack substantially. They added that oestrogen replacement therapy in post-menopausal women and regular low doses of aspirin in men could have important adjunctive roles. The latest evidence (Department of Health, 1995a) on the benefits of regular, light alcohol consumption for middle-aged men and women would indicate that this strategy should be considered to be as effective as those mentioned at the beginning of this paragraph.

This book will focus only on the dietary components which act as behavioural risk factors. In the Round Table Model shown in the colour section, the fourth ring relates only to dietary factors. For the sake of clarity and simplicity, all dietary factors discussed in the text are illustrated in this Model. The evidence for some effects on physiological risk factors is much greater for some than for others (see Chapter 6).

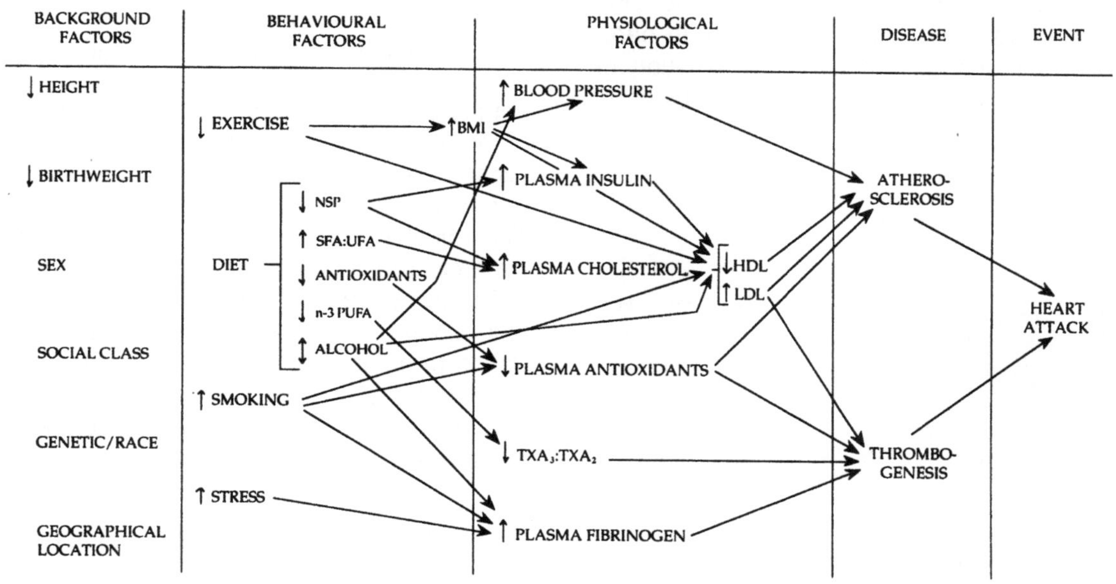

Figure 1.10 Inter-relationship between behavioural and physiological risk factors. NSP, non-starch polysaccharides; SFA, saturated fatty acids; UFA, unsaturated fatty acids; PUFA, polyunsaturated fatty acids; BMI, body mass index; TX, thromboxane; HDL, high density lipoprotein; LDL, low density lipoprotein.

2

PATHOLOGY – EVENTS LEADING TO CORONARY HEART DISEASE

(See the inner ring of the Round Table Model in the colour section)

The heart is a muscular pump which contracts regularly to keep blood flowing through the body's extensive network of blood vessels. The heart muscle itself receives blood via the coronary arteries.

If these become blocked, blood supply to the heart muscle is impaired and the tissue suffers from a lack of oxygen and nutrients. This can lead to chest pain on exertion (angina) and irregularities in the heart beat (arrhythmia). In severe cases it can cause the heart to stop beating and is fatal.

The coronary arteries may become blocked by a blood clot in conjunction with the previous deposition of various materials forming a fibrous plaque on the inner arterial walls (atherosclerosis).

The events leading to arterial blockage can be described simply as a three-stage process and are represented by three sections in the inner ring in the Round Table Model (see colour section):

1. Injury to coronary arteries.
2. Atherosclerosis or build-up of the fibrous plaque.
3. Thrombosis and heart attack.

These three stages are described in the following sections, although the sequence of events leading to atherosclerosis is not fully understood. In particular there is much debate over the initiation of atherosclerosis (Addis and Park, 1988; Fuster *et al.*, 1992).

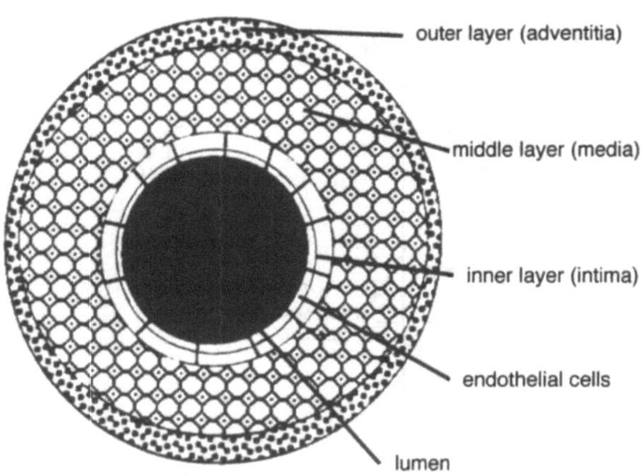

Figure 2.1 Diagrammatic cross-section through a normal artery.

2.1 INJURY TO CORONARY ARTERIES

The endothelial cells lining the lumen of the arteries (Figure 2.1) are able to respond to normal wear and tear. Minor lesions are repaired by deposition of small blood cells called platelets and the formation of small blood clots.

However, continual minor injuries to the endothelial cells can lead to more severe damage which affects the underlying layers of cells, the intima of the arterial wall. Minor injuries are caused by disturbances in the pattern of blood flow and possibly by bacterial injury. They are exacerbated by factors such as increased levels of damaged lipid particles and free radicals derived from cigarette smoke.

Once the layer of endothelial cells is damaged, the platelets stick to the surface of the damaged cells and the plasma constituents can pass more easily through to the deeper layers of the artery walls. A growth factor derived from the platelets causes smooth muscle cells in one of these layers, the media, to multiply and move outwards into the intima.

The outcome is a thickening of the intima due to the production of collagen from the smooth muscle cells, and deposition of cellular material from the walls of dead cells (Figure 2.2).

It is thought that the initial arterial injury in atherosclerosis can be caused by the excessive uptake of damaged lipid particles by macrophages in the artery wall. This also stimulates further multiplication and movement of smooth muscle cells and exacerbates thickening of the intimal layer. The initial injury can also be caused by hemodynamic turbulence and by bacterial injury.

The initial damage might then be exacerbated by high blood pressure (BP) which increases the infiltration of components of blood into the artery wall. An increased tendency for platelets to aggregate and inflammation will also exacerbate the effects of any damage.

2.2 FIBROUS PLAQUE FORMATION

Fibrous plaque is formed at the site of injury by deposition of oxidized blood lipids, platelets, and strands of protein, fibrin, which form a mesh.

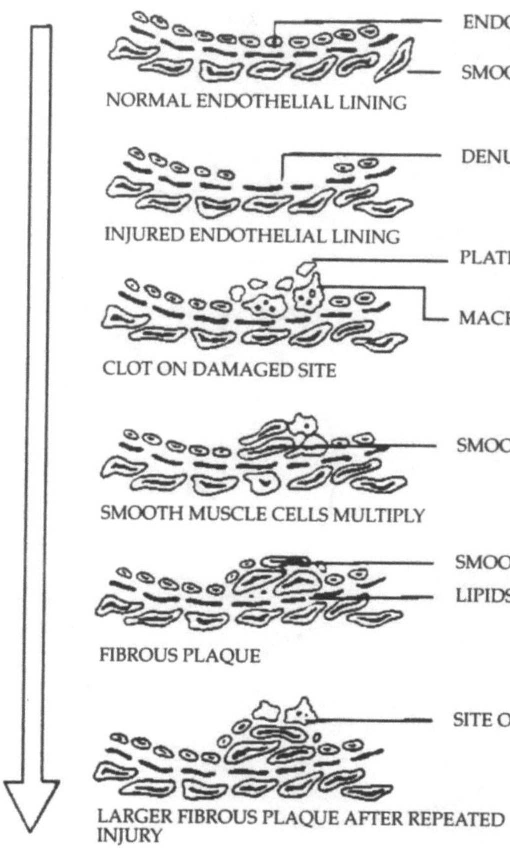

Figure 2.2 Diagram showing the progression and formation of fibrous plaques.

2.2.1 Lipoprotein metabolism

Figure 2.3 shows essential stages in the metabolism of lipoproteins. Digestion of dietary fat and cholesterol results in the absorption of fatty acids which are then re-assembled into triglycerides and cholesterol esters and packaged into chylomicron (CM) particles for their transport in the circulation. CMs are the largest of the lipoprotein particles (i.e. molecules which contain apoproteins as well as lipids to increase their hydrophilic nature) and the TG they contain is susceptible to hydrolysis by lipoprotein lipase (LPL) so that fatty acids are delivered to cells and smaller chylomicron remnants (CM-R) are formed.

Very low density lipoproteins (VLDL), like chylomicrons, contain predominantly TG and their function is to transport the TGs which are made in the liver or gut. The low density lipoproteins (LDL) are derived from VLDL by a series of steps which remove TGs and their role is to deliver cholesterol to the cells in a well-regulated process such that the cells only take up as much cholesterol as they need. High density lipoproteins (HDL) carry excess cholesterol away from the peripheral cells to the liver, a process known as reverse cholesterol transport.

2.2.2 Lipid oxidation and deposition

Damage to the layer of endothelial cells attracts a certain type of circulating white blood cell (monocyte) to the site of injury. Monocytes ingest bacteria and other foreign particles. Once they have passed through the arterial wall they are called macrophages (Figure 2.4).

Macrophages are cells of the immune system whose function is to absorb foreign or toxic components. They have 'scavenger' receptors which allow them to recognize and remove oxidized lipid particles which may be toxic to cells in the area. Macrophages play a major role in fibrous plaque formation by interacting with damaged (usually oxidized) LDL particles which transport lipids, such as cholesterol, in the blood.

The protein component of the lipoprotein particle (the apoprotein) helps to solubilize the lipid and to target it to cell receptors. Apoprotein B (apoB), the major protein of LDL, is usually 'recognized' by the normal LDL receptor and is taken up by cells that require cholesterol (see Figure 2.3). However, polyunsaturated fatty acids (PUFA) within the lipids in LDL particles can become oxidized, causing changes to the structure of apoB such that the protein is not recognized by the cell receptors and is

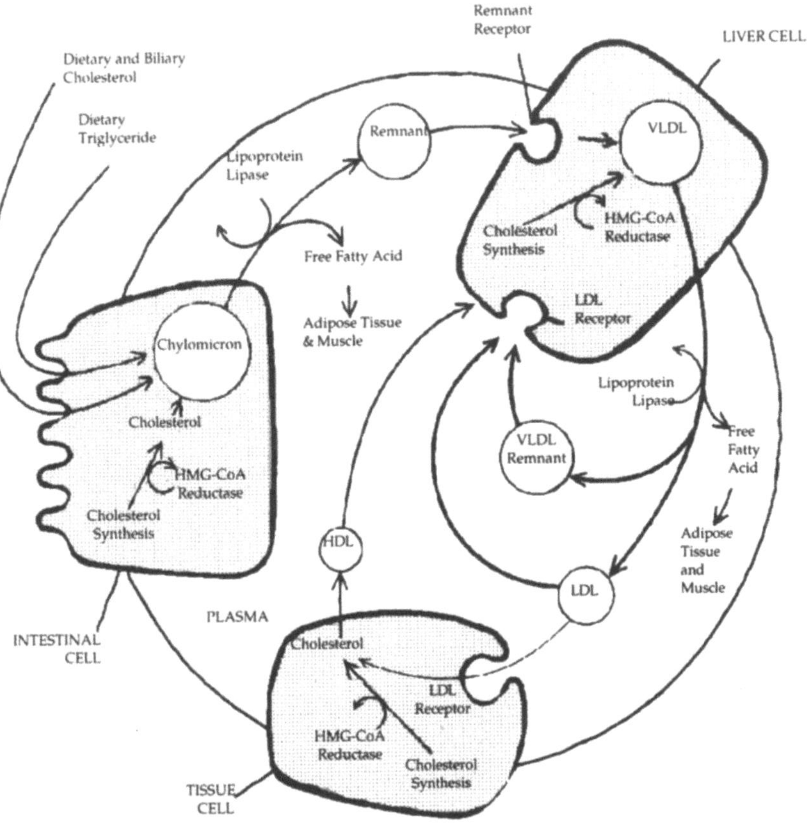

Figure 2.3 The metabolism of lipoproteins. HMG-CoA, 3-hydroxy-3-methylglutaryl coenzyme A; VLDL, very low density lipoprotein; LDL, low density lipoprotein; HDL, high density lipoprotein.

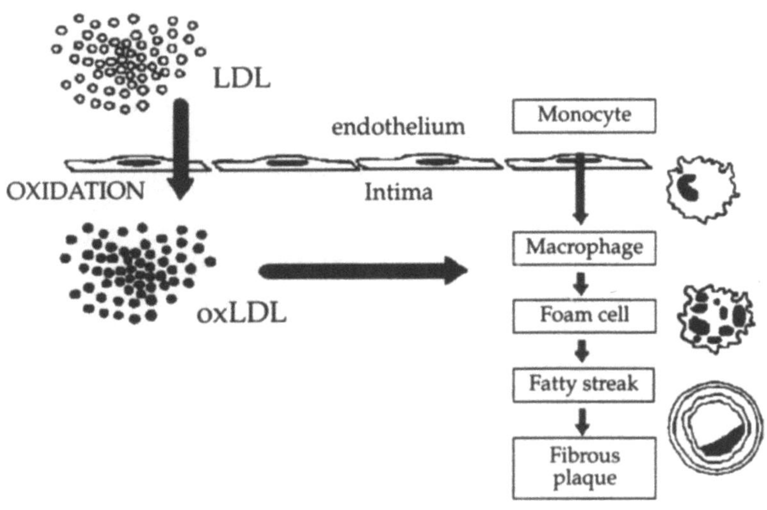

Figure 2.4 Role of oxidized LDL in the formation of fibrous plaque. LDL, low density lipoprotein; oxLDL, oxidized LDL. (Source: Brown 1992.)

taken up by macrophages. Macrophages can become overloaded with oxidized LDL and form 'foam cells'.

The foam cells ultimately die and deposit their entrapped lipid on the walls of the arteries. Foam cells are possibly one of the earliest recognizable lesions of atherosclerosis (see Figure 2.4).

2.2.3 Involvement of the blood clotting system

Damage to the arterial wall also triggers the blood clotting mechanism.

Various elements in the blood associate to form a minor thrombus that seals a wound. The repair system is complex because it needs to be assembled at the site of the damage and to be removed when the repair has been effected. If the repair system were not under strict control there would be constant danger that unwanted and dangerous thrombi could be formed or, at the other extreme, that the slightest cut could lead to continual bleeding, as occurs in haemophilia.

Wound healing is brought about by:

- platelet aggregation – clumping of platelets to form larger aggregates; and
- formation of a mesh composed of strands of an insoluble protein, fibrin.

Damage to arterial endothelial cells triggers the wound healing process, leading to the formation of platelet aggregates. Platelets are cell fragments with an outer membrane made of phospholipids containing PUFA and various proteins including receptors for collagen.

Platelets are activated when collagen or other agents which initiate aggregation interact with the surface receptors. The PUFA, arachidonic acid, is present in the membrane phospholipids of the platelets and is then released by the enzyme phospholipase A2 and converted into thromboxane which stimulates aggregation. Thromboxane also

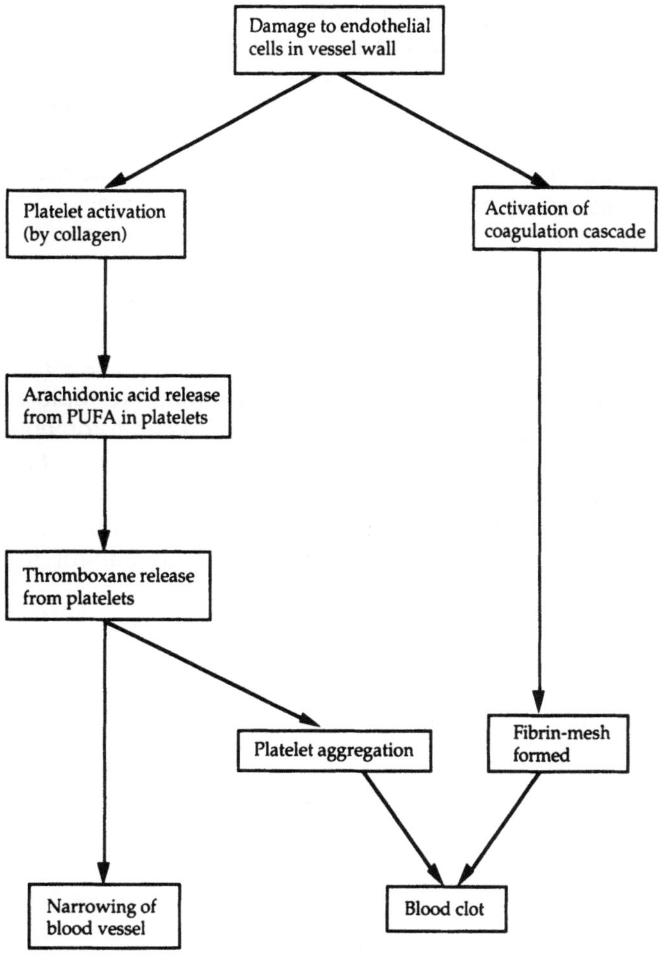

Figure 2.6 Mechanisms to reduce blood loss from a wound. PUFA, polyunsaturated fatty acids.

causes the blood vessel to narrow (vasoconstriction). This reduces the amount of blood lost through the wound.

Fibrin is normally present in the blood in its soluble, inactive form, fibrinogen. Transformation of fibrinogen to fibrin by the enzyme thrombin is the final stage of a long sequence of transformations known as the coagulation cascade, in which many 'inactive' components or factors are changed to their active form.

Undamaged endothelial surfaces of the blood vessels inhibit induction of this cascade. When they are damaged a specific cell membrane protein called tissue factor is exposed. This interacts with Factor VII present in the blood and triggers the cascade that produces a fibrin mesh (Figure 2.5).

This traps red blood cells and clumps of platelets which together form a wound-sealing clot or thrombus (Figure 2.6). Formation of a thrombus over the site of injury can also become incorporated into the growing fibrous plaque.

Continual thickening of the fibrous plaque results in gradual narrowing of the artery. This causes disturbances in blood flow, increasing the tendency for

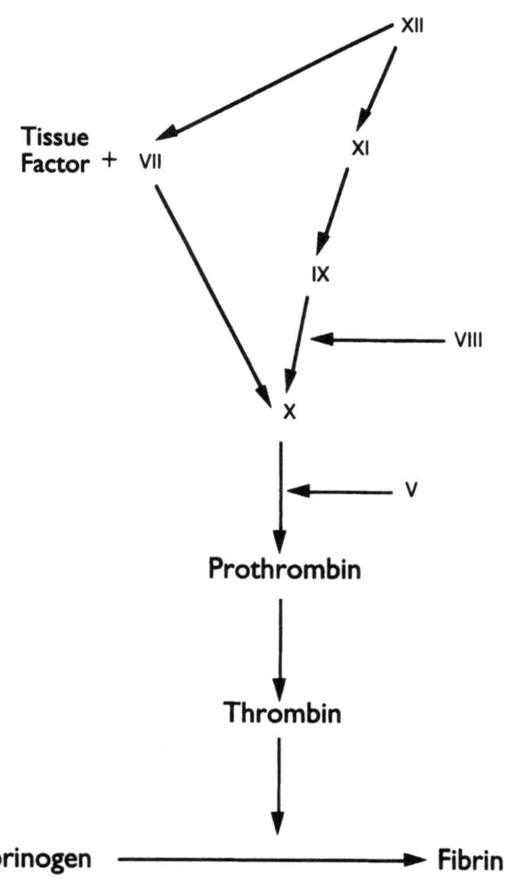

Figure 2.5 The coagulation cascade converting fibrinogen to fibrin. V, VII, VIII, IX, X, XI, XII are clotting factors.

further damage and growth of the fibrous plaque.

Fibrinolysis is the process by which blood clots are dissolved and removed from the circulation. The dissolution of fibrin in a clot is mediated by the enzyme, plasmin, and fibrin serves as a cofactor for the activation of plasmin. Inhibitors of fibrinolysis act by preventing the activation of plasmin.

2.3 THROMBOSIS AND HEART ATTACK

When the fibrous plaque becomes unstable, it becomes mechanically weak and tends to rupture. This can trigger formation of a major thrombus, through platelet aggregation and the coagulation cascade, which blocks the artery.

Another important consideration in thrombosis risk is the balance of factors which control the relaxation of the underlying smooth muscle cells in the arteries. Blood platelets release substances in response to injury which stimulate the endothelial cells to produce vasodilatory prostaglandins; these can oppose the actions of other vasoconstricting prostaglandins. The endothelial cells themselves produce a vasodilator called endothelium-derived relaxing factor (EDRF) which is now known to be the gas, nitric oxide (NO). Therefore, if the ratio of vasoconstrictor substances to vasodilator substances is increased, the risk of thrombosis is higher.

Formation of a large thrombus in an artery already narrowed by fibrous plaque can completely obstruct the blood flow to the heart. In severe cases, a lack of oxygen supply to a vital part of the heart muscle causes a heart attack or myocardial infarction.

3

PHYSIOLOGICAL RISK FACTORS

(See Figure 3.1 and the second ring of the Round Table Model in the colour section)

3.1 INCREASED BLOOD PRESSURE

High BP exacerbates initial damage to arterial walls by increasing the infiltration of blood components.

Increased BP has been shown to predict development of CHD in a number of prospective studies. Men in the top quintile of diastolic BP (>92 mmHg) when originally screened for entry into the Multiple Risk Factor Intervention Trial (MRFIT) had 2.4 times the risk of dying from CHD as those in the lowest quintile (<76 mmHg). The relative risk between the highest and the lowest quintiles was greater in younger age groups; the greatest difference was 5.4 for people aged 35 to 39 years (Kannel *et al.*, 1986).

However, a recent intervention drug trial of 16 000 people in Glasgow with uncomplicated high BP, found no significant effect on the subsequent incidence of heart attacks. Intervention did however reduce the number of strokes by nearly half (MRC Working Party, 1988).

3.2 INCREASED LIPID OXIDATION

There is sufficient evidence now to regard lipid oxidation as an important risk factor for CHD (Brown, 1992; Regenstrom *et al.*, 1992; Salonen *et al.*, 1992a; Witzum, 1994).

Preventing oxidation of fatty acids in LDL particles is an important step in preventing the initial arterial injury (Steinberg *et al.*, 1989).

Many factors affect the potential of LDL to

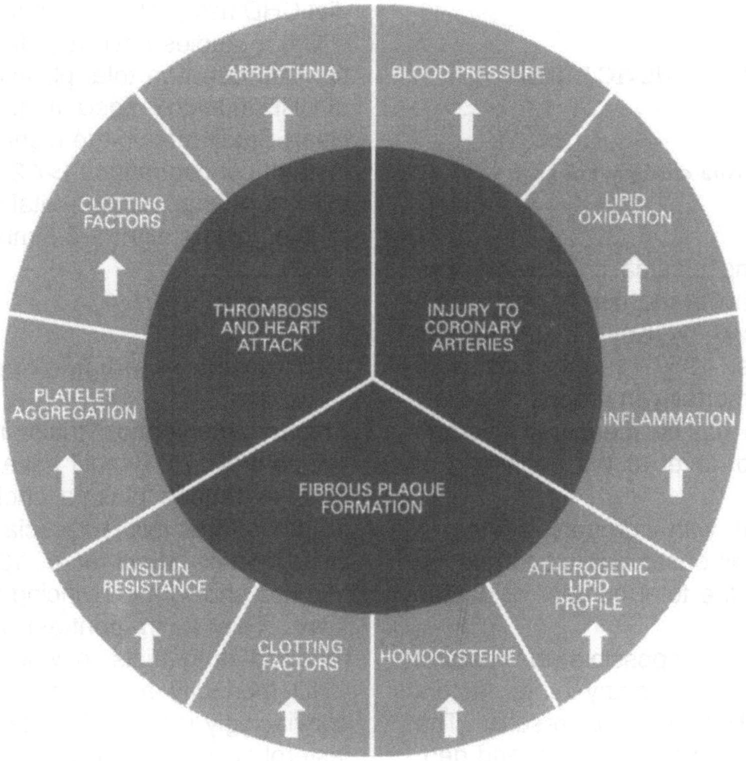

Figure 3.1 The inner and second rings of the Round Table Model showing the physiological risk factors (second ring) which influence the three stages of heart disease shown in the inner ring. Some risk factors influence more than one stage and this is explained in the text.

become oxidized but three of the most important are :

- oxidizability of fatty acids in the LDL particle
- the amount of pro-oxidants present
- the availability of antioxidants.

PUFA are more susceptible to oxidation than saturated fatty acids (SFA) because they contain more than one double bond in the fatty acid chain (Hodgson *et al.*, 1993).

Oxidation occurs by free radical attack, which means that a chain reaction is triggered, attacking all PUFA molecules in the vicinity. The free radicals, which are molecular species with unpaired electrons, can be produced naturally in the body by phagocytic cells and are present in tobacco smoke and industrial pollutants. Free radical attack can be catalysed by the presence of pro-oxidants such as free ions of copper and iron but can be inhibited by antioxidant molecules which can donate an electron to terminate the reaction without themselves becoming free radicals (British Nutrition Foundation, 1991).

3.3 INCREASED INFLAMMATION

Inflammation of the injured area of arterial wall exacerbates the effect of the damage and, in some cases, can initiate it.

3.4 INCREASED ATHEROGENIC LIPID PROFILE

3.4.1 Evidence for plasma cholesterol as a risk factor

Evidence that circulating plasma cholesterol concentration is correlated with the risk of death from CHD was first produced by Keys in the Seven Countries Study (Keys, 1957, 1980). This work examined subsequent mortality in groups of mainly rural middle-aged men having measured average plasma total cholesterol level at the beginning of the study.

A striking correlation with coronary deaths in each group or cohort was observed. In contrast, no relation was seen with the total number of deaths from all causes.

Data of this type are impossible to interpret unequivocally in view of the many other factors which might have influenced the results. The groups of men came from varied cultural and geographic regions and the association of coronary deaths over a period of years with the initial plasma cholesterol concentration cannot be assumed to be causal without substantial additional evidence.

Subsequent studies concentrated on individuals rather than groups of men in specific locations, and from defined racial, cultural and age groups. The most comprehensive study has been the Framingham Study (Kannel and Gordon, 1970). This long-term prospective study of a small American town has yielded a wealth of data on a particular population.

Many measurements including plasma cholesterol were made on men and women of various ages and causes of death, including CHD, were recorded over various time periods

The results suggested that in men under 65 years, coronary mortality is higher in those with higher plasma cholesterol levels. In men within the range of cholesterol levels 4.0 to 6.2 mmol/l (150–250 mg/100 ml) the curve of CHD deaths against plasma cholesterol level is shallow and flattens with increasing age. The slope of the total mortality curve decreases with age and there is an inverse relationship with plasma cholesterol levels for men over 55 years. Of course, although relative risk might decrease with increased age, the absolute risk will still increase and the 'lives saved' are as high as in the younger age group.

For women (not shown) the observed relationships were more straightforward but with significant numbers of coronary deaths only in the older age groups. Equations have now been produced, based on the Framingham data, which help to predict CHD risk (Anderson *et al.*, 1991).

Other studies have also found a curvilinear relationship between total plasma cholesterol and risk of CHD in middle-aged men. In the British Regional Heart Study men in the highest fifth of plasma cholesterol concentrations (>7.2 mmol/l) had 3.5 times the risk of fatal and non-fatal CHD events than men in the lowest fifth (<5.5 mmol/l) (Pocock *et al.*, 1989).

3.4.2 Problems with lowering plasma cholesterol

Primary intervention trials in those with plasma cholesterol >7.5 mmol/l have shown that it is possible to reduce plasma cholesterol using diet or drugs and that this is associated with a reduction in CHD mortality (Frick *et al.*, 1987). However, no diet trial has shown a convincing reduction in total mortality. This is in contrast to the most recently reported drug trials in which plasma cholesterol, CHD morbidity and total mortality have all been convincingly reduced by 'statins' which inhibit cholesterol synthesis (Oliver, 1995).

A meta-analysis of six primary prevention trials (Muldoon *et al.*, 1990) has shown that reducing plasma cholesterol levels in middle-aged men led to a significant reduction in CHD mortality. There

LEGEND TO THE ROUND TABLE MODEL

- The inner ring represents the three pathological events (see Chapter 2) in chronological sequence – injury to coronary arteries, fibrous plaque formation, thrombosis and heart attack.
- The second ring represents the physiological risk factors (see Chapter 3) and relates them to the three stages of heart disease as determined by the pathological events.
- The third ring represents the uncontrollable factors (see Chapter 4) which are background factors influencing all the physiological risk factors. In some cases, they will also influence the dietary (other controllable) factors.
- The fourth ring represents the dietary factors which affect the different physiological risk factors (see Chapter 6). Other controllable factors such as smoking and exercise are not illustrated in this model, but must be considered to influence the physiological risk factors directly and also through their relationship with the dietary factors.

The segments relating to each stage of heart disease should be interpreted in the following way:

- Dietary factor X positively influences physiological risk factor Y which increases the likelihood of the occurrence of pathological event Z.
- e.g. severe obesity increases blood pressure which increases the likelihood of injury to the coronary artery.
- e.g. high saturated fatty acids intake increase LDL-cholesterol formation which has an adverse effect on the atherogenic lipid profile and thus increases the likelihood of fibrous plaque formation.

The outside rings therefore represent undesirable dietary factors because they determine undesirable physiological risk factors.

For the sake of clarity and simplicity, all dietary factors discussed in the text are illustrated in this Model. The evidence for some effects on physiological risk factors is much greater for some than for others (see Chapter 6).

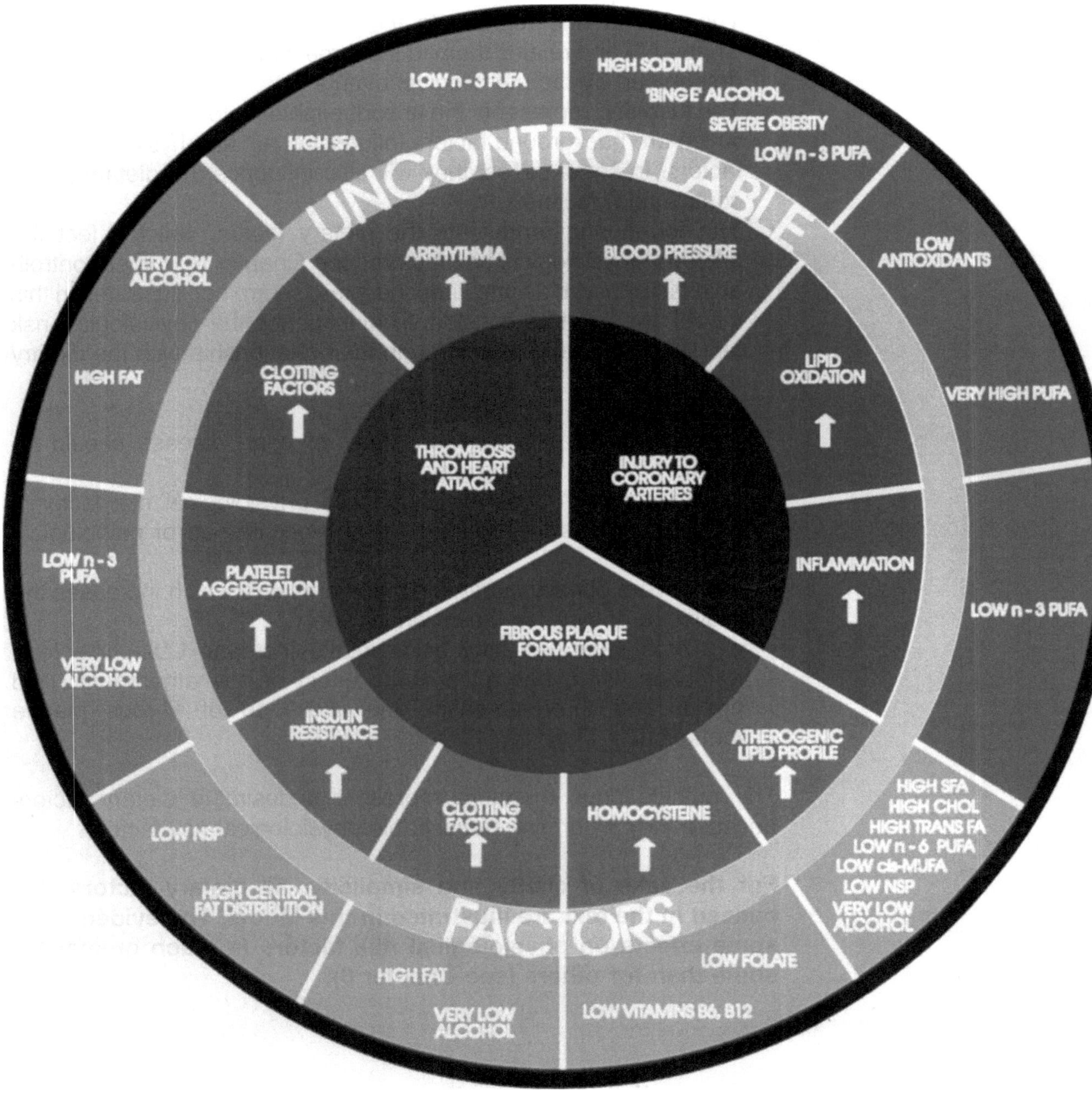

UNCONTROLLABLE
FACTORS
THROMBOSIS AND HEART ATTACK
INJURY TO CORONARY ARTERIES
FIBROUS PLAQUE FORMATION
ARRHYTHMIA
BLOOD PRESSURE
LIPID OXIDATION
INFLAMMATION
ATHEROGENIC LIPID PROFILE
HOMOCYSTEINE
CLOTTING FACTORS
INSULIN RESISTANCE
PLATELET AGGREGATION
CLOTTING FACTORS
LOW n - 3 PUFA
HIGH SFA
HIGH SODIUM
'BINGE' ALCOHOL
SEVERE OBESITY
LOW n - 3 PUFA
LOW ANTIOXIDANTS
VERY HIGH PUFA
LOW n - 3 PUFA
HIGH SFA
HIGH CHOL
HIGH TRANS FA
LOW n - 6 PUFA
LOW cis-MUFA
LOW NSP
VERY LOW ALCOHOL
LOW FOLATE
LOW VITAMINS B6, B12
HIGH FAT
VERY LOW ALCOHOL
HIGH CENTRAL FAT DISTRIBUTION
LOW NSP
LOW n - 3 PUFA
VERY LOW ALCOHOL
HIGH FAT
VERY LOW ALCOHOL

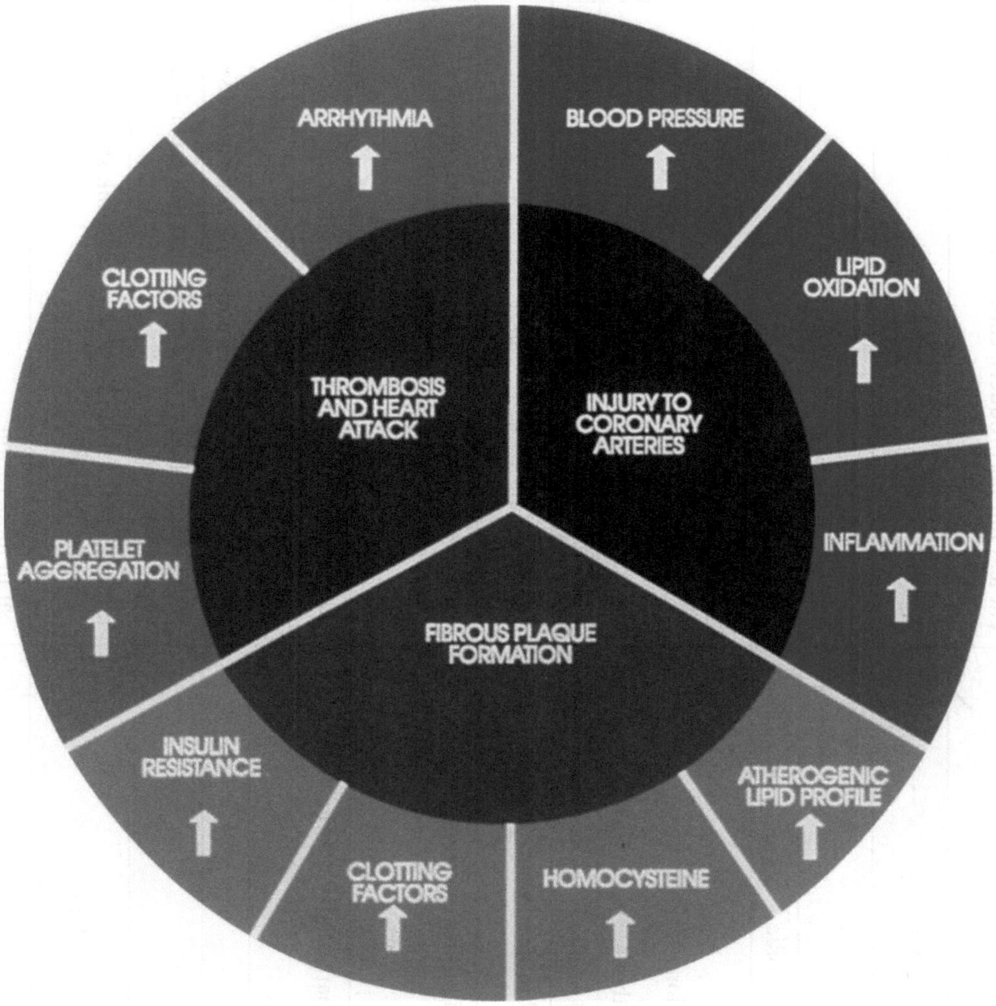
ARRHYTHMIA
BLOOD PRESSURE
LIPID OXIDATION
INFLAMMATION
ATHEROGENIC LIPID PROFILE
HOMOCYSTEINE
CLOTTING FACTORS
INSULIN RESISTANCE
PLATELET AGGREGATION
CLOTTING FACTORS
THROMBOSIS AND HEART ATTACK
INJURY TO CORONARY ARTERIES
FIBROUS PLAQUE FORMATION

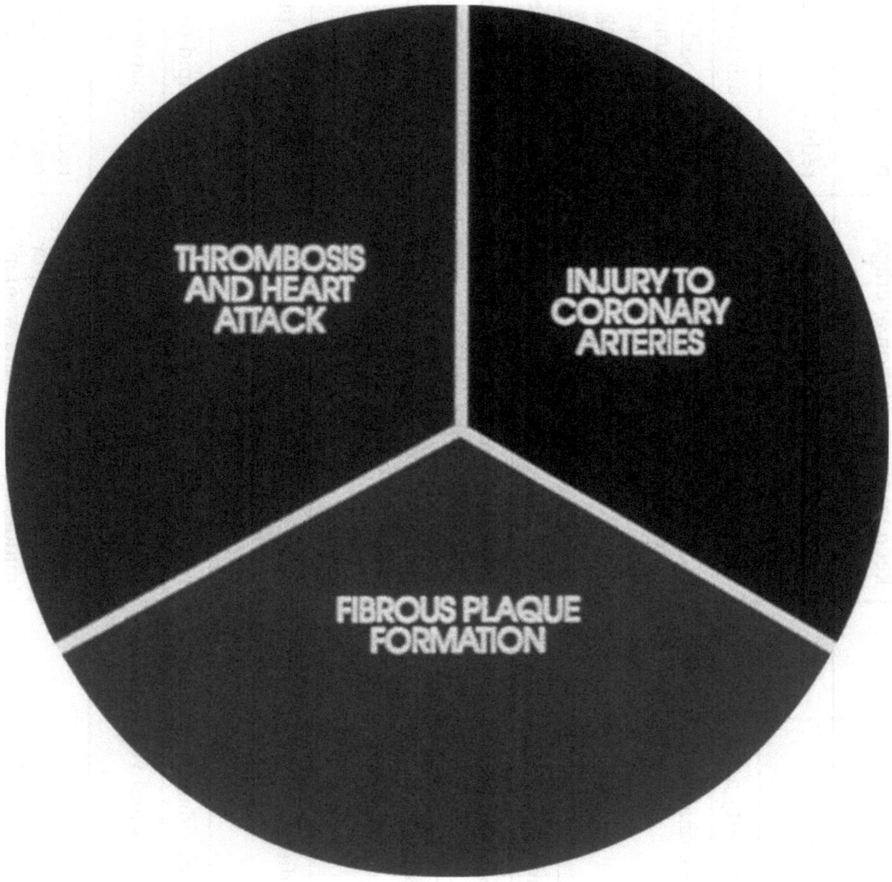
THROMBOSIS AND HEART ATTACK
INJURY TO CORONARY ARTERIES
FIBROUS PLAQUE FORMATION

SUMMARY OF CHANGES REQUIRED TO FOOD AND DRINK

Dietary factor	**Recommendation**	**Interaction with physiological risk factor**	**Changes required to food and drink**
Total fat	reduce from 40% to population average of 33% TDE[1,3]	reduce atherogenic lipid profile	eat less full-fat products, choose low-fat options
SFA	reduce from 16% to population average of 10% TDE[1,3]	reduce atherogenic lipid profile	eat less full-fat products, choose low-fat options
n-6 PUFA	keep up to population average of 6% TDE[1,3]	reduce atherogenic lipid profile	
cis-MUFA	keep up to population average of 12% TDE[1,3]	reduce atherogenic lipid profile	
trans fatty acids	keep down to 2% TDE[1,3]	reduce atherogenic lipid profile	
Long-chain n-3 PUFA	increase from 0.1 g per day to population average of 0.2 g per day[3]	reduce blood pressure reduce inflammation reduce platelet aggregation reduce clotting factors reduce severity of arrhythmia	eat at least one portion oil-rich fish per week
Cholesterol	keep low[1,3]	reduce atherogenic lipid profile	
NSP (soluble)	increase from 12 g to population average 18 g per day[1]	reduce atherogenic lipid profile; reduce insulin resistance	eat more fruit, vegetables and wholegrain cereals
Starches	increase from 24% to population average of 37% TDE, including starches, intrinsic and milk sugars[1]	reduce atherogenic lipid profile (indirectly)	eat more potatoes, rice, pasta, bread and cereals
Sodium	reduce population average intakes from 9 g salt per day to 6 g per day[3]	reduce blood pressure, particularly the rise with age	add less salt to food; eat less high-salt food
Antioxidant nutrients	increase[2]	reduce lipid oxidation	eat more fruit, vegetables and wholegrain cereals
Folates and vitamins B_6 and B_{12}	increase[2]	reduce plasma homocysteine	eat more fortified cereals and bread and green-leafy vegetables
Alcohol	avoid 'binge drinking'[4]; keep low, regular alcohol intake for middle-aged men and women[4];	reduce blood pressure reduce plasma LDL, increase HDL reduce clotting factors	middle aged men and women who drink should have 1–2 units per day[4]
Energy	maintain body weight within desirable range[3], particularly if high central fat distribution[2].	reduce insulin resistance	eat in moderation

TDE, total dietary energy; LDL, low density lipoprotein; SFA, saturated fatty acids; PUFA, polyunsaturated fatty acids; MUFA, monounsaturated fatty acids; Lp(a), lipoprotein(a); NSP, non starch polysaccharides

[1] Department of Health, 1991 [3] Department of Health, 1994
[2] Consensus view [4] Department of Health, 1995

was no reduction in total mortality, as there was an equivalent and significant rise in deaths from other causes, notably accident, violence and suicide.

This is not necessarily a causal relationship, although previous clinical studies have found low plasma cholesterol measurements in criminals, those with 'poorly internalized social norms', and those who exhibit violent or aggressive conduct. The effect is also more likely to be seen when cholesterol is lowered by drug rather than diet (Davey Smith and Pekkanen, 1992; Davey Smith *et al.*, 1993).

There have also been suggestions that a low plasma cholesterol concentration is associated with an increased risk of cancer. It has been argued, however, that a low plasma cholesterol concentration may be a result of a pre-existing undiagnosed cancer and some studies have tried to take this into account in their analyses by excluding people who developed cancer within 4 years of cholesterol measurement (Isles *et al.*, 1989). The meta-analysis by Muldoon *et al.* (1990) found a non-significant increase in cancer mortality in the intervention groups.

A meta-analysis by Law *et al.* (1994) found that excess mortality associated with levels of serum cholesterol <5 mmol/l was not seen in studies of employed men, but was restricted to community cohorts who are likely to include larger numbers with pre-existing illness.

The problems of having a low cholesterol *per se* and of acquiring a low cholesterol through lowering cholesterol were reviewed and summarized in the 1994 CRG Report (Department of Health, 1994).

'Some, but not all, prospective studies have shown an association between low plasma cholesterol at initial examination and increased total and non-cardiovascular mortality at follow-up, and trials of cholesterol-lowering drugs have found increased mortality in the intervention groups. The reasons for these two observations may be different. In prospective studies at least some of the increased mortality associated with low cholesterol can be attributed to pre-existing disease or confounding. Increased non-cardiovascular mortality is not found in populations with low average concentrations of cholesterol. There is no evidence that lifelong low plasma cholesterol, rather than more short-term reduction of plasma cholesterol in middle age, is associated with adverse effects'.

3.4.3 Raised low density/high density lipoprotein cholesterol ratio

Raised LDL-cholesterol has been positively associated with CHD in numerous prospective studies. The relationship is seen most clearly in individuals with familial type II hyperlipidaemia. This condition is caused by a genetic defect in the synthesis of LDL receptors and is characterized by high circulating levels of LDL-cholesterol.

Plasma concentrations of LDL-cholesterol in heterozygotes (10–15 mmol/l) are up to three times those found in the general population and are increased by up to six-fold in homozygotes. Heterozygotes below the age of 60 years are around 25 times more likely to suffer a CHD event than the general population. Homozygotes usually suffer a heart attack before the age of 20 years.

For the levels more commonly found in the general population, a 10-year prospective study of men with no evidence of CHD at the beginning of the trial found that the risk of dying from CHD was 2.7 times higher for men with LDL-cholesterol levels >4.1 mmol/l than for men with levels <3.4 mmol/l (Pekkanen *et al.*, 1990).

The British Regional Heart Study confirmed previous prospective studies in showing that a low concentration of HDL-cholesterol was also a risk factor for CHD. The risk of CHD was twice as high in men with the lowest levels of HDL-cholesterol (<0.93 mmol/l) compared with men with the highest levels (>1.33 mmol/l) (Pocock *et al.*, 1989).

It has been suggested that, due to their opposing effects, the ratio of LDL to HDL-cholesterol may be the most important determinant of risk. Gordon *et al.* (1989) have proposed, on the basis of four prospective studies, that an LDL/HDL-cholesterol ratio >3.5 leads to increased risk of CHD.

The most recent equations to predict CHD risk based on the data from the Framingham study recognize the superiority of the ratio of total cholesterol to high density lipoprotein (HDL) cholesterol (Anderson *et al.* 1991).

3.4.4 UK cholesterol levels

Despite widespread health promotion campaigns in the UK, average population plasma cholesterol levels have remained remarkably constant over the past 15 or so years. A survey carried out in 1986 (Gregory *et al.*, 1990) found that mean plasma cholesterol level in men and women (aged 16 to 64 years) was 5.8 mmol/l.

A recent national survey of nearly 17 000 English adults carried out in late 1993 again recorded mean plasma cholesterol levels at 5.8 mmol/l in men and 5.9 mmol/l in women (Bennett *et al.*, 1995). Older women tended to have higher mean levels than men of the same age; the converse was true among those aged between 25 to 44.

Average plasma cholesterol levels are higher in the UK than in many other parts of the world. For example average levels in China are 3.3 mmol/l

(Peto *et al.*, 1989). When the majority of the population has high plasma cholesterol, other factors are possibly more important in determining relative risk.

This may explain why no regional differences in plasma cholesterol concentrations are seen in the UK despite regional differences in CHD mortality rates, and why plasma cholesterol concentrations are higher for people with non-manual occupations, although their mortality rates are lower than those with manual occupations.

3.4.5 Increased plasma lipoprotein(a) levels

Lipoprotein (a) [Lp(a)] is similar in lipid composition to LDL but is slightly larger and more dense because it contains an additional protein moiety, apoproteinA [apoA] as well as apoB. ApoA is similar in composition to plasminogen (an important component of the fibrinolytic pathway) and Lp(a) is believed to be one of the molecules which might link atherosclerosis and thrombogenesis, although the evidence for its relationship to lipoprotein levels is greater than that relating to its thrombogenic potential (Lawn, 1992).

Both case-control and prospective studies have shown that an increased level of Lp(a) is correlated with CHD independently of other risk factors (Ridker *et al.*, 1993) and Lp(a) levels are particularly high in people with familial hypercholesterolaemia and diabetes.

Like LDL, the Lp(a) molecule is prone to oxidation and may be taken up by macrophages to form foam cells with the usual consequences of arterial injury and plaque formation (see Chapter 2) (Berg, 1991).

It was originally thought that plasma levels of Lp(a) were under genetic control and not influenced by dietary factors, but there is now limited evidence to show that some dietary components can influence Lp(a) (see Chapter 6).

3.4.6 Increased postprandial lipaemia

Although high fasting triglyceride (TG) levels are not considered an independent risk factor for CHD, there is increasing evidence that TG levels in the postprandial state could provide an important determinant of the risk of CHD (the TG intolerance hypothesis) (see Figures 2.3 and 3.2).

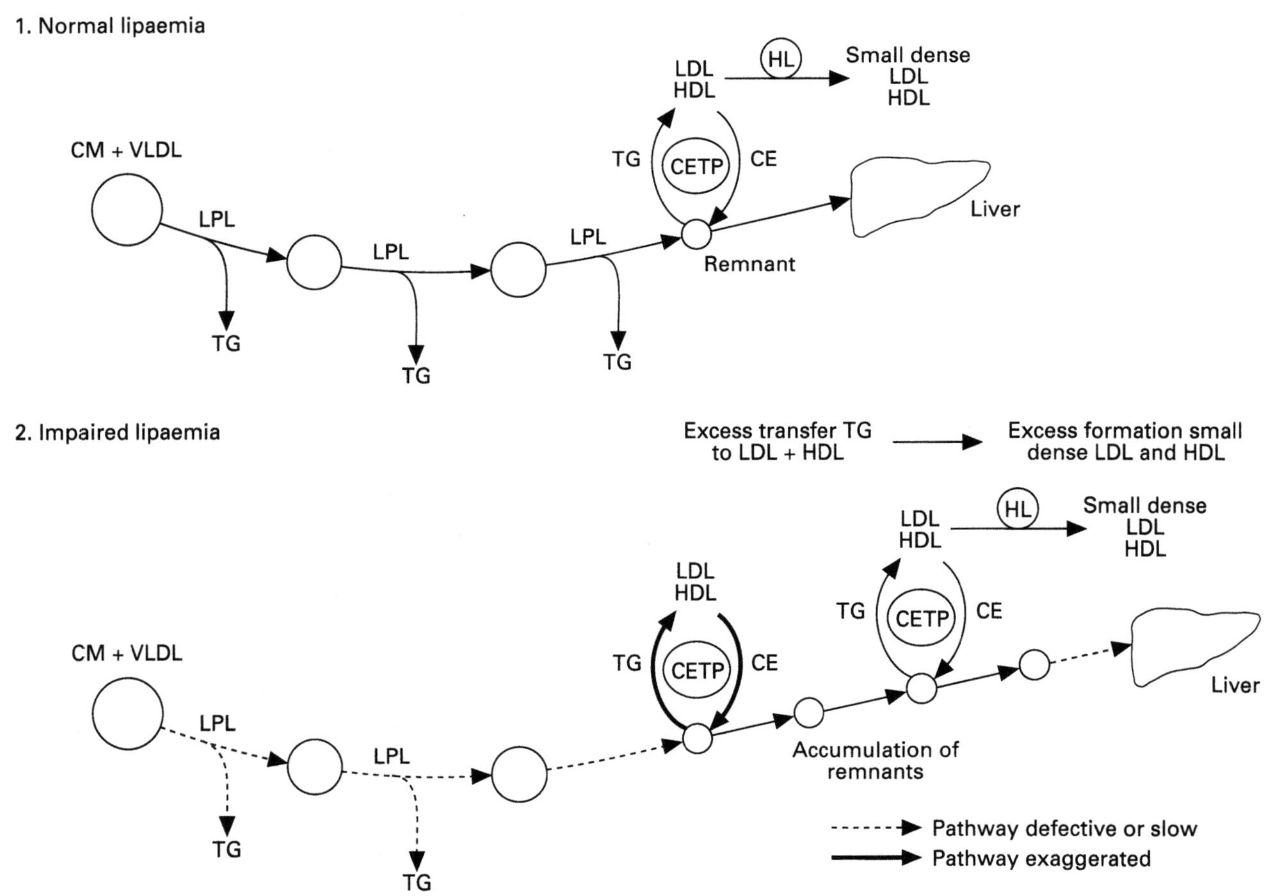

Figure 3.2 Relationship between postprandial lipaemia and formation of small, dense HDL and LDL. LPL, lipoprotein lipase; HL, hepatic lipase; CETP, cholesterol ester transfer protein. (With acknowledgement to C. H. Williams.)

Any physiological challenge to the normal fasting state of the lipid transport system (e.g. ingestion of a fat-containing meal) will lead to postprandial lipaemia, which is thought to be the time period between food ingestion and approximately 6 to 8 hours thereafter. So because we eat fairly regularly throughout the day, postprandial lipaemia is the characteristic condition of most people for 12 to 18 hours of the day.

The first indication that low density lipoprotein cholesterol (LDL) and also chylomicron remnants (CM-R), when enriched by dietary cholesterol, can be taken up by the arterial wall was reported by Zilversmit (1979). Human monocytes and macrophages possess receptors specific for CM-R which are different to the LDL receptor and this is how the CM-R are transported through the arterial wall. The possibility that chylomicrons which play a major role in dietary triglyceride (TG) metabolism, may be potentially atherogenic, has led to the postprandial lipoprotein hypothesis (Patsch, 1987).

Abnormal TG response to a meal results in an exaggerated increase in postprandial plasma TG levels and/or an extension of the time that the TG particles stay in the circulation.

An increase in postprandial plasma TG levels could result in an increase in TG transport from CM and VLDL to LDL and HDL through the action of cholesterol ester transfer protein (CETP). The same enzyme will reciprocally transfer cholesterol from LDL and HDL to CM and VLDL. As a consequence, CM-R will become cholesterol-enriched and LDL and HDL will become TG enriched. These particles are susceptible to hydrolysis by hepatic lipase and so they become smaller and denser. All of these lipoprotein particles increase CHD risk because they are poorly removed by liver receptors and are therefore free to be taken up by the arterial wall.

There are also adverse consequences for the reverse cholesterol transport system (i.e. HDL) which is normally responsible for removing atherogenic LDL from the circulation. The decreased HDL-cholesterol concentrations result from increased hydrolysis of the TG within the lipoprotein particles by lipoprotein lipase (LPL). These effects and their consequences are summarized in Table 3.1.

Possible mechanisms which can affect the extent and duration of postprandial lipaemia are linked with the activities of the enzymes CETP and LPL. Decreased CETP activity has been associated with increased CHD risk, and decreased LPL activity results in greater postprandial lipaemia because of slow clearance of TGs and prolonged residence time of CMs and their remnants in the circulation. Mutations of the LPL gene have been linked with pronounced postprandial lipaemia, but interest also exists in the effects of dietary fatty acid composition on postprandial lipaemia and LPL activity for preventive reasons (see Chapter 6).

3.5 INCREASED PLASMA HOMOCYSTEINE LEVELS

McCully (1969) was the first to propose that high plasma levels of total homocysteine (Hcy) resulted in severe and premature atherosclerosis, because he had noticed the widespread incidence of vascular disease in infants who had died from homocysteinuria. Now that simple and reliable methods for measuring plasma homocysteine have

Table 3.1 Effect and consequences of a disorder in postprandial lipaemia*

Effect	Consequences
Increase in plasma TG levels and increased residence in circulation, by relative decrease in LPL synthesis and/or activity and relative increase of substrate for CETP activity	Increased transfer of TG to HDL and LDL, and of CE to CM and VLDL
Formation of cholesterol-enriched and TG-poor chylomicron remnants	Increased uptake into arterial wall
Formation of TG-enriched LDL, TG-enriched CE-poor HDL and increased HL activity in liver, acting on TG in LDL and HDL particles	Increased small and dense LDL and HDL formation
Formation of small dense LDL particles	Increased uptake into arterial wall
Increased formation of small dense HDL particles	Less reverse cholesterol transport

TG, triglyceride; HDL, high density lipoprotein; LDL, low density lipoprotein; LPL, lipoprotein lipase; CD, cholesteryl ester; CM, chylomicron; VLDL, very low density lipoprotein; CETP, cholesteryl ester transfer protein; HL, hepatic lipase.
*From Zampelas (1994).

been developed, the hypothesis that increased levels of homocysteine may play an important role in CHD has been advanced once more.

The prospective Physicians Health Study (Stampfer *et al.*, 1992) showed that the 271 men who later had myocardial infarctions (MI) had significantly higher levels of Hcy than matched controls who remained free of infarction. Those with homocysteine levels in the highest 5% had three times the adjusted risk of MI. A prospective study in middle-aged men in the British Regional Heart Study also suggested that Hcy was a strong and independent risk factor for stroke (Perry *et al.*, 1995)

In a cross-sectional study of more than 1000 subjects from the original Framingham Heart Study, Selhub *et al.* (1995) found associations between the degree of narrowing (stenosis) of the carotid artery and Hcy levels and also with the intakes of the B vitamins involved in homocysteine metabolism. The men and women within the highest quartile of Hcy levels were twice as likely as the people in the lowest quartile to show greater degrees of stenosis.

In the same year, Den Heijer *et al.* (1995) reported from a case-control study of 185 cases and 220 control subjects that increased Hcy was associated with recurrent venous thrombosis (odds ratio = 3.1) and suggested that moderately high levels of plasma homocysteine were associated with greater likelihood of plaque rupture, leading to thrombus formation and myocardial infarction

A meta-analysis of 27 studies relating Hcy level to arteriosclerotic vascular disease concluded that a total of 10% of the population's CHD risk appears attributable to Hcy and that a 5 μmol/l increment in Hcy elevates CHD risk by as much as increases in plasma cholesterol of 0.5 mmol/l (Boushey *et al.*, 1995).

Studies on the mechanism of action of homocysteine suggest that an increased level of plasma homocysteine is probably a physiological risk factor for increased thrombosis and arterial injury as well as for increased risk of fibrous plaque formation (Ubbink, 1995), but it has been placed in this section of the Round Table Model since the risk factor was originally associated with atherogenesis.

3.6 INCREASED BLOOD CLOTTING FACTORS

3.6.1 Increased plasma fibrinogen levels

High fibrinogen levels may contribute to atherosclerosis, increase blood viscosity and influence the amount of fibrin formed when coagulation is initiated. Fibrinogen is also an important cofactor in platelet aggregation. High levels can therefore be a risk factor which increase both fibrous plaque formation and the likelihood of thrombus formation.

Plasma fibrinogen levels appear to be the strongest biochemical index of CVD and a number of prospective studies have found that plasma fibrinogen levels are strongly associated with the subsequent incidence of CHD.

In one such study, men in the highest third of plasma fibrinogen levels had three times the risk of heart attack (fatal or non-fatal) during the following 5 years compared with the men in the lowest third. In the same study, men with the highest serum cholesterol concentration had twice the risk of men with the lowest values (Meade *et al.*, 1986).

The main determinant of plasma fibrinogen levels is smoking. Plasma fibrinogen levels fall after smoking ceases and reach levels found in non-smokers after about 7 years. They have also been correlated, independently of smoking, with levels of reported job dissatisfaction (Markowe, 1985). This interesting finding may help to explain the relationship between CHD and the most elusive component of CHD – stress.

Plasma fibrinogen levels do not appear to be determined by diet to any great extent, and neither is there a suitable fibrinogen-lowering drug. A primary intervention trial has not yet, therefore, been possible.

3.6.2 Increased Factor VII

The results of the Northwick Park Heart Study (Meade *et al.*, 1986) showed that Factor VII coagulant activity, as well as plasma fibrinogen concentration, was a strong predictor of CHD.

3.6.3 Decreased fibrinolysis

Several cross-sectional studies have indicated an association between low fibrinolytic activity and CHD and more recently Meade *et al.* (1993) showed in a prospective study that low fibrinolytic activity is a strong independent predictor of CHD, especially in young men.

3.7 INCREASED INSULIN RESISTANCE

3.7.1 Evidence for increased insulin resistance being a CHD risk factor

A non-insulin-dependent diabetic has twice the risk of CHD as someone without diabetes. A number of prospective studies have found that elevated plasma insulin levels are associated with a subsequent increased risk of CHD in normal men (Cambien *et al.*, 1986).

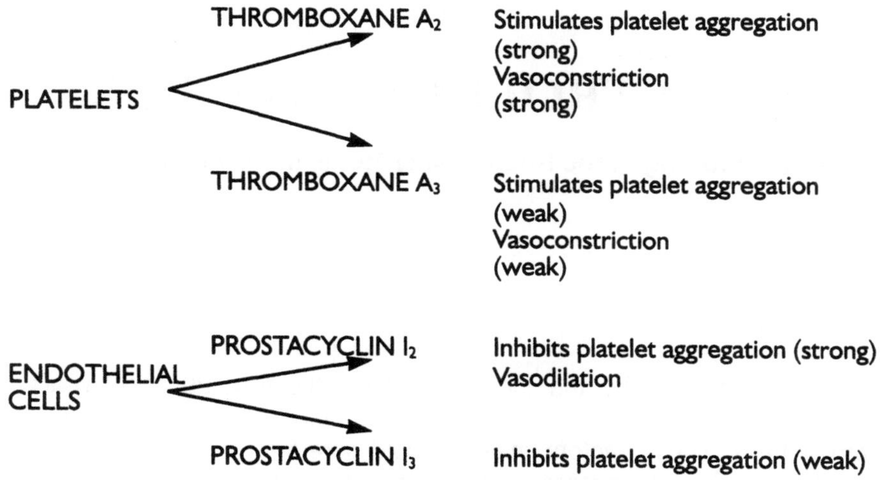

Figure 3.3 Factors affecting platelet aggregation and the diameter of arteries.

Other studies have found that healthy people with high plasma insulin levels have multiple risk factors for CHD, including higher fasting plasma triglyceride levels (an associated risk factor), lower plasma HDL-cholesterol levels and higher BP than those with normal insulin levels. Plasma glucose levels measured after drinking a standard amount of glucose, were higher in volunteers with high plasma insulin levels than in those with normal insulin levels.

This resistance to the action of insulin and the subsequent hyperinsulinaemia may be the cause of increased plasma triglyceride and low HDL-cholesterol levels. This may also explain the clustering of multiple risk factors in some people, the so-called Syndrome X (Zavaroni *et al.*, 1989).

This pattern of metabolic abnormalities has also been observed in Bangladeshis and has been suggested as the cause of the high CHD rates in Southern Asians generally.

3.7.2 Mechanism of action?

It is not yet certain that insulin resistance and the consequent raised levels of insulin cause CHD or whether they are just accompanying facets. It is suggested, however, that insulin increases arterial wall lipid synthesis and smooth muscle cell proliferation (Department of Health, 1994). Raised levels of insulin are also thought to stimulate VLDL formation by the liver with consequential increases in LDL formation.

3.8 INCREASED PLATELET AGGREGATION

The factors involved in formation of a thrombus or blood clot (thrombogenesis) are not fully understood. Essentially, it depends on the balance between the factors favouring platelet aggregation and narrowing of the artery, and factors that counterbalance them (Figure 3.3) (see British Nutrition Foundation, 1992a).

Thromboxanes, released from platelets, favour platelet aggregation and vasoconstriction. Prostacyclins, released from endothelial cells in the arterial wall, inhibit platelet aggregation and cause the arteries to relax (vasodilation). The various types of thromboxanes and prostacyclins differ in the strength of their effects.

An imbalance in the synthesis of these compounds could favour thrombogenesis and increase the chances of a heart attack.

3.9 INCREASED ARRHYTHMIA

Diseased heart muscle is susceptible to bouts of irregular electrical activity (arrhythmia). This causes the heart beat to become irregular which can influence the outcome and severity of a heart attack.

4

UNCONTROLLABLE FACTORS

(See the third ring of the Round Table Model in the colour section)

Factors which cannot be controlled by the individual include genetic make-up, age, sex, race and possibly early growth pattern. These factors may act by influencing both behavioural patterns and the physiological risk factors which produce conditions favouring the development of CHD. Though the mechanisms of action have not yet been fully determined, some clues have been found (British Nutrition Foundation, 1992b).

It is possible that some of the detrimental effects of uncontrollable factors can be counteracted by changes in behavioural factors such as taking more exercise, stopping smoking, controlling stress and eating a well-balanced diet. Characterization of the factors, however, will allow individuals with high risk to be identified and appropriate preventative measures adopted.

4.1 EFFECTS OF AGE, SEX AND RACE ON CORONARY HEART DISEASE

4.1.1 Effects of age and sex

As a baby grows, fatty streaks which might be precursors to fibrous plaque formation, can be found near the sites where the arteries branch. This is probably due to the disturbance in blood flow at these sites which results in short-term lipid deposition. These lesions subsequently disappear until the adolescent growth spurt when they reappear.

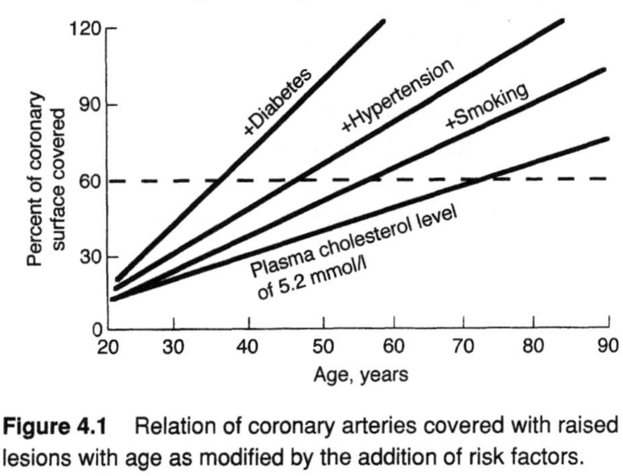

Figure 4.1 Relation of coronary arteries covered with raised lesions with age as modified by the addition of risk factors. (Source: Grundy, 1988.)

Over the next 20 or 30 years more established fibrous plaques develop, often taking the form of a lipid core with a fibrous cap. These may occur at the same sites as the fatty streaks in some people. It is probable that ageing on its own has little effect on CHD and merely represents the cumulative effects of other risk factors such as increased plasma cholesterol levels and BP.

It has been suggested that a critical stage is reached when more than half of the coronary surface is covered by atherosclerotic lesions and that in the absence of any risk factors (i.e. normal BP, normal plasma cholesterol levels), this stage is reached at about 70 years. Figure 4.1 shows how the accumulation of risk factors would cause this critical stage to be reached at an earlier age.

In men and women the death rate from CHD rises steeply with increasing age (Table 4.1). Up to the age of 45 years the number of deaths from CHD in UK men is about five times that in women.

The death rate from CHD in women (deaths per 100 000 population) lags behind that for men by about 10 years. Death rates in women increase approximately six-fold between the ages of 35–44 and 45–54 years, i.e. before and after the menopause. This is similar to the increase in male death rates between 25–34 and 35–44 years.

Although the number of deaths from CHD in women over 75 years is greater than men of the same age, the proportion of deaths due to CHD is lower because the female population at this age is larger than the male population.

Deaths from CHD as a proportion of total deaths in each age group are also higher in men than women at all ages, although the difference between the sexes decreases with increasing age (Figure 4.2).

The relative protection afforded to premenopausal women has been attributed to:

- higher levels of HDL-cholesterol;
- lower iron stores;
- peripheral, rather than central, fat distribution.

These factors may all be explained by effects of the sex hormone oestrogen. One study in Sweden

Table 4.1 Annual death rates from CHD and as a proportion of total deaths in the UK – the effect of age and sex

	Male			Female		
Age (years)	CHD deaths	CHD deaths/ 100 000 population	% of deaths	CHD deaths	CHD deaths/ 100 000 population	% of deaths
25–34	189	5	5	28	1	2
35–44	1 436	37	21	249	6	5
45–54	5 898	189	37	1 135	36	12
55–64	17 591	610	38	5 845	191	21
65–74	32 099	1 441	35	17 908	639	28
75+	39 950	3 064	28	53 443	2 097	25

Source: WHO, 1989.

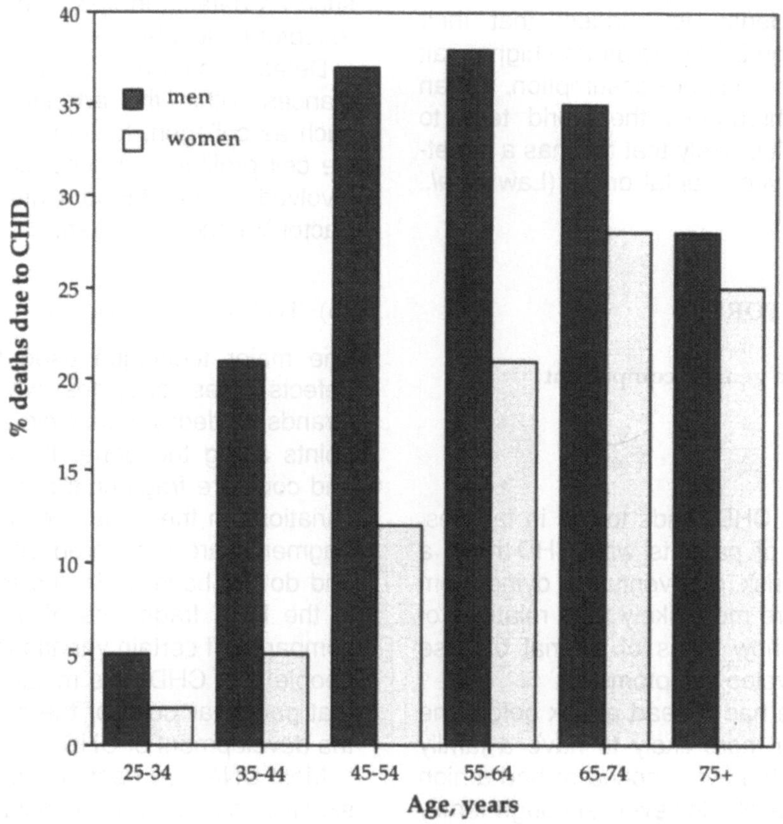

Figure 4.2 Deaths from CHD as a proportion of all deaths for different age and sex groups. (Source: WHO, 1989.)

found that the sex difference in CHD rates was completely explained by differences in fat distribution (Lapidus *et al.*, 1984).

4.1.2 Racial differences (see also Chapter 1)

(a) Asians

Asians living in the UK but originating from Gujarat, Punjab, Bangladesh, Pakistan and Southern India have rates of CHD 40% higher than the UK national average (McKeigue *et al.*, 1991). Asian migrants in other parts of the world also have relatively high rates.

The difference in rates of CHD mortality between Asians and white Caucasians in the UK cannot be explained by differences in diet, plasma cholesterol levels or smoking habits (McKeigue *et al.*, 1985). Most surveys suggest that smoking rates and plasma cholesterol levels are lower among Asians than the general population. Furthermore, their intakes of saturated fatty acids (SFA) and total fat are lower than the national average.

One possible reason for excess CHD rates among Asians is the increased prevalence of non-insulin-dependent diabetes mellitus, which in some Asian communities in London is four times the national average. The insulin resistance syndrome and central fat distribution are also more common among Asians (McKeigue *et al.*, 1991) than Europeans (see Chapter 3).

(b) Afro-Caribbeans

Afro-Caribbeans in the UK have lower rates of CHD mortality than the UK national average but higher rates of stroke and high BP. It is not known why they have lower rates of CHD mortality despite high rates of diabetes and high BP. The prevalence of diabetes is almost as high as in Asians, but insulin resistance or central obesity is less common than in European men (McKeigue *et al.*, 1991).

There is no evidence to suggest that their increased rates of high BP are related to higher salt intakes or increased alcohol consumption. Urban black populations throughout the world tend to have higher BP and it is likely that this has a genetic rather than an environmental origin (Law *et al.*, 1991).

4.2 GENETIC FACTORS

4.2.1 Evidence for a genetic component (Berg, 1983)

(a) Family studies

It is well known that CHD tends to run in families. The close relatives of patients with CHD have a five- to seven-fold risk of eventually dying from heart disease and are more likely than relatives of healthy people to show signs of arterial disease even before they develop symptoms.

Patients who have had a heart attack before the age of 55 years are more likely to have a family history of CHD than to have smoked or had a high plasma cholesterol level. However, although family studies could indicate a genetic component of a disease, they could also indicate the importance of shared environmental factors such as diet.

(b) Twin studies

Studies of identical and non-identical twins can provide stronger evidence of genetic predisposition than family studies. Both share the same environment, but only identical twins share the same genes.

If a twin has CHD there is a 65% chance that an identical twin will have CHD, but only a 25% chance that a non-identical twin will have CHD. If CHD occurs before the age of 60 there is an 83% chance that an identical twin will have CHD but the risk does not increase further for a non-identical twin (Chamberlain and Galton, 1990).

4.2.2 Possible mechanisms for a genetic component

(a) A range of candidate genes

If a family tendency to CHD is due to a genetic component, which of the 1.4 million genes in the human genome could be involved?

Because of the multifactorial nature of CHD there is the possibility for a wide range of gene defects to be involved. These could lead to abnormalities in lipid transport and lipid uptake into arterial walls such as defects in lipoprotein molecules and their receptor molecules.

Defects could also affect genes coding for substances within the arterial wall, macromolecules such as collagen, factors involved in smooth muscle cell proliferation, local cell growth, and factors involved in the blood clotting cascade such as Factor VII and fibrinogen.

(b) Technical approaches

The major technique used to determine genetic defects uses enzymes which are able to cut strands of deoxyribonucleic acid (DNA) at specific points along the gene. It is possible to separate and compare fragments of the gene which contain variations in the genetic code. If these small DNA fragments are compared between people who do and do not have CHD, the frequency of variations in the DNA fragments of the two groups can be compared. If certain variations are more frequent in people with CHD, this might imply that variation at that particular point of the gene is associated with the development of CHD.

Most DNA fragments have no currently identified significance but they can act as genetic markers for major genes found nearby.

The detection of such markers might lead to the eventual identification of the mutations responsible for the inherited basis of the disease.

Although molecular biological techniques can be very precise, the precision of the diagnosis of heart disease is not always as good. Patients might be grouped together on the basis of clinical symptoms, but these symptoms might have arisen for different reasons.

(c) Low density lipoprotein receptor

Familial hypercholesterolaemia affects about 1 in 500 among Caucasian populations. It is characterized by high levels of LDL-cholesterol in the blood and premature CHD, and is due to a single gene defect involving the LDL receptor.

Although this particular gene defect occurs too infrequently to account for the common forms of CHD, it is possible that other variations within the gene for the LDL receptor may lead to protein variants of the receptor which could modify LDL binding and promote fibrous plaque formation.

(d) Apoprotein B

The apoproteins are responsible for transporting lipids around the body. ApoB is one of the proteins of LDL which transports lipids and cholesterol to the tissues (see Chapter 2). The human apoB gene is found on chromosome 2. The complete amino acid sequence of apoB is known and the particular region of the protein has been identified which binds to the normal LDL receptor.

A rare single gene mutation has been reported which impairs binding of the LDL apoB to its receptor. This leads to the clinical condition known as familial defective apoB100 characterized by raised levels of LDL in the blood and premature CHD. Like the defect in the LDL receptor which leads to familial hypercholesterolaemia, it is a very rare mutation and cannot account for the widespread occurrence of premature CHD seen in the general population.

(e) Lipoprotein lipase

Analysis of DNA from people with premature atherosclerosis has shown a difference in the gene coding for lipoprotein lipase (LPL) on chromosome 8. LPL is the enzyme responsible for the uptake of triglycerides into cells. This gene difference could lead to raised levels of triglycerides in the blood which are associated with increased risk of CHD although they do not appear to be an independent risk factor.

(f) Enzymes of homocysteine metabolism

The best evidence for a candidate gene which can contribute to high plasma levels of homocysteine (Hcy) is the gene controlling the production of the enzyme 5,10-methylenetetrahydrofolate reductase (MTHFR). This enzyme catalyses the reaction that leads to the formation of the predominant circulatory form of folate (5-methyltetrahydrofolate) which is the carbon donor for the re-methylation of homocysteine to form methionine.

The existence of a thermolabile form of MTHFR with reduced activity which could lead to increased Hcy levels has been reported in patients with CHD. This variant has been observed in the homozygous form in about 5% of the general population, in about 17% of patients with CHD and in about 28% of patients with premature vascular disease who had homocysteinuria (Kang *et al.*, 1991). Whether nutritional deficiency of folic acid alone will raise Hcy levels or whether this response is limited to individuals who are genetically predisposed to developing high Hcy levels is uncertain (Boushey *et al.* 1995).

4.2.3 Future developments

CHD is a very complex disease process. In spite of overwhelming evidence that CHD has a strong genetic component, it will be some time before the major genes, which have defects causing a propensity to CHD, can be identified.

Inconsistencies found between genetic studies may reflect the heterogeneity of CHD. Selecting people at random to find the 'normal' background may also produce a gene-pool which is too mixed for large differences to emerge. In future it will be important to ensure that cases and controls come from the same gene pool, i.e. belong to the same ethnic subgroups and preferably originate from the same geographical locality.

It has been suggested (Berg, 1991) that genetic influences may determine an individual's ability to adapt to behavioural modification of the physiological risk factors as well as determining the actual levels of the risk factors themselves. Genetic combinations as well as interactions between genes and their environment must be considered if the complexities of CHD are to be unravelled.

4.3 POSSIBLE INFANT ORIGINS OF CORONARY HEART DISEASE

4.3.1 Effect of height

Factors acting in early life might have consequences for the later risk of CHD (see Barker, 1991 for review). It has been known for some time that short people are more likely than tall people to die from CHD. Height is largely determined by growth in early childhood.

The Whitehall study (Marmot *et al.*, 1978) found that height was inversely related to CHD mortality. Men less than 5 feet 6 inches (1.68 m) tall have 1.5 times the risk of CHD than men over 6 feet (1.83 m). Height was also closely correlated with employment grade in this study.

4.3.2 Effect of disproportionate fetal growth

It has been proposed more recently that CHD is associated with specific patterns of disproportionate fetal growth that result from fetal undernutrition in mid- to late gestation (Barker, 1994), and also that these early changes programme later disease.

This hypothesis is supported by animal studies which show that undernutrition before birth programmes persisting changes in a variety of metabolic, physiological and structural processes. In addition, studies in humans have indicated increased rates of CHD in men and women whose weight at birth fell within the lower end of the normal range and who were also thin or short at birth, or small in relation to the size of the placenta.

The fetal period is a period of rapid growth, characterized by cell division. Different tissues have different 'critical periods' during which their growth is particularly intensive. Nutrients and oxygen are needed for this process and if supply is limited, the rate of growth slows. Cell division is particularly affected in those tissues growing rapidly. The slowing of growth may either be a direct effect or secondary to a fall in concentration of growth factors or hormones, e.g. insulin and growth hormone. The outcome of a period of undernutrition will depend on which tissues are growing rapidly at that particular time.

Barker (1995a) has suggested that undernutrition in humans, as demonstrated long ago in pigs by Widdowson (1974), may permanently reduce the number of cells in particular organs. It may also permanently change the distribution of cell types, the patterns of hormonal secretion, metabolic activity and organ structure. The hypothesis that these changes can be translated into pathology in later life is a new, though perhaps unsurprising, concept. Short periods of undernutrition *in utero* in animals have been shown to result in persisting changes in blood pressure, cholesterol metabolism, insulin response to glucose, and other effects on metabolic, endocrine and immune function.

However, CHD incidence is not higher in proportionately small babies, such as those born to mothers in developing countries. In such infants, small size may be a downward adjustment in growth rate geared to match the low nutrient availability experience right from the outset of pregnancy. Slower growth would put less demand on nutrient supplies.

A total of 16 000 men and women born in Hertfordshire between 1911 and 1930 have now been traced by Barker's research group. Detailed records of these individuals' birth weights and dimensions and their progress during the first year of life have been compared with current information about these people. Death rates from CHD in adulthood fall progressively as birth weight of the individuals rises from 5.5 lb (2500 g) to 9.5 lb (4310 g). Data from Sheffield have indicated that it is the individuals who were small at birth because they had failed to grow well, rather than those who were born prematurely, that are at increased risk to disease. These trends are paralleled by effects on major risk factors for CHD.

The prevalence of non-insulin-dependent diabetes was three times greater in men who weighed 5.5 lb at birth compared with those weighing 9.5 lb. This finding has also been demonstrated with other populations in Britain and also in Sweden and in the USA. Trends in raised blood pressure with low birth weight are also apparent. Evidence from different populations from around the world shows that children who are small at birth are more likely to have raised blood pressure and signs of an inability to respond to an oral glucose challenge.

Paneth and Susser (1995) and Bartley *et al.* (1994) have suggested that the associations Barker has reported can be explained by bias due to differential survival, selective migration and confounding variables linked with lifestyle during adulthood. However, Barker believes that the evidence from various studies, which have included populations in which child mortality is low, counters these claims.

Further studies by Barker's group, using records from Preston, have shown that thinness at birth, measured by a low ponderal index (birth weight ÷ length^3) is associated with insulin resistance syndrome, characterized by impaired glucose tolerance, raised blood pressure and disturbed lipid metabolism in adult life which can lead to CHD. This has been confirmed in a Swedish study, and is supported by observations in India.

Thin babies lack muscle as well as fat, and muscle is the main peripheral site of action of insulin, which has a key role in stimulating cell division in fetal life. Barker suggests that a baby that is born thin has been undernourished at some time during mid- to late gestation, and this has resulted in the muscles becoming insulin resistant. However, growth of the brain is spared at the expense of muscle development.

Evidence for programming of serum cholesterol and blood clotting factors comes from the Sheffield records. Babies at risk of CHD in later life are those born with disproportionate dimensions – a short body in relation to the size of the head. This kind of growth pattern is thought to relate to undernutrition in late gestation, and an adaptation by the fetus to divert oxygenated blood away from the trunk in order to sustain the brain. This compromises linear growth and growth of the abdominal viscera.

The Sheffield records included abdominal girth, and a reduction in this measurement at birth was predictive of raised serum LDL-cholesterol concentration in adult life. The differences in concentration of LDL-cholesterol across the range of girth measurements was large, and was equivalent statistically to a 30% difference in CHD mortality. An interpretation of this finding is that a small girth reflects impaired liver growth and consequent reprogramming of liver metabolism.

Interference with growth at any stage of gestation seems to be associated with a persisting increase in blood pressure, which is found in people who were thin or short or proportionately small at birth. A total of 21 studies have reported an association between low birth weight and subsequently raised blood pressure. The ratio of birth weight to placental weight also predicts blood pressure. There is evidence that women who are anaemic, who exercise heavily while pregnant, or who live at high altitude develop large placentas, possibly to extract more nutrients. Barker suggests that possible mechanisms include persisting changes in vascular structure, including loss of elasticity in vessel walls, and effects of glucocorticoid hormones (as evidenced from animal studies).

These observations are consistent with an effect of early development on an individual's later risk of CHD, which may be related to nutritional factors including the method of infant feeding. The effects on CHD mortality seem at least partly to be mediated through recognized risk factors. They appear to act independently of, and in addition to, environmental effects, such as diet and obesity later in life.

Barker and colleagues are now investigating some of the mechanisms that can account for these epidemiological observations. An animal model has demonstrated that reductions in protein content of the pregnant rat can programme the functioning of a number of tissue systems in adulthood. Metabolic studies in humans using indirect calorimetry have shown that middle-aged women who were small at birth oxidize less of an oral glucose load than those who were relatively large at birth. Further studies with stable isotopes have demonstrated reduced rates of glycolysis in skeletal muscle. This predisposition to impaired glucose tolerance, possibly as part of a glucose-sparing effect, may result from a resetting of major hormonal axes influencing growth and metabolism.

Barker (1995b) has concluded that CHD 'arises not primarily from external forces but from the body's self-organization, homeostatic settings of enzyme activity, cell receptors, and hormonal feedback, which are established in response to undernutrition *in utero* and lead eventually to premature death'.

4.4 EFFECT OF STRESS ON CORONARY HEART DISEASE

The scientific basis for the belief that CHD is linked to stress is not as firm as often thought, mainly because of the problem of defining stress and deciding how much is too much. It is also debatable whether stress should be included as an uncontrollable factor. One accepted definition of the type of stress that leads to CHD is that stress is an overload of external demands, more often referred to as psychosocial factors. Personal, home, social, work and environmental factors can all be included in this category and justify the inclusion of stress as an uncontrollable factor in some instances. The reader is referred to the recent review by Brunner (1995) for further consideration of stress and CHD.

4.5 INFECTIOUS AGENTS AS A CAUSE OF CORONARY HEART DISEASE

Many studies have reported that evidence of past infection with organisms such as *Helicobacter pylori* which commonly affects the stomach, and *Chlamydia pneumoniae* which commonly affects the lungs, is significantly associated with increased risk of CHD. On the basis of a cross-sectional study of almost 400 white middle-aged men living in London, Patel *et al.* (1995) have suggested that these chronic infections, when accompanied by persistent inflammation, can increase blood levels of acute phase reactants, including fibrinogen, which are physiological risk factors for CHD.

5

DIETARY FACTORS

The effect of different dietary factors on the physiological risk factors for CHD will be explained in Chapter 6. This chapter provides some basic facts about the relevant nutrients.

5.1 DIETARY FATS

5.1.1 Chemistry

The main dietary lipids (fats) are triglycerides which contain three molecules of fatty acids on a backbone molecule of glycerol. Fatty acids consist of chains of carbon atoms with hydrogen atoms attached to them, with an acid carboxyl group (COOH) at one end and a methyl (CH_3) group at the other end of the molecule.

Saturated fatty acids (SFA) have two hydrogen atoms attached to each carbon atom. Unsaturated fatty acids contain one or more double bonds which occur when two hydrogen atoms on a pair of adjacent carbon atoms are absent. Monounsaturated fatty acids (MUFA) have a single double bond and polyunsaturated fatty acids (PUFA) have two or more double bonds (Figure 5.1).

A double bond can adopt one of two geometrical configurations, called *cis* and *trans*. *Cis* double bonds are more commonly found in lipids, although *trans* bonds occur in a few of the fatty acids of ruminant fats, plant leaf lipids and some seed oils. *trans* bonds are also produced during the 'hardening' of vegetable oils.

A shorthand nomenclature for fatty acids gives the length of the carbon chain, followed by a colon and the number of double bonds. Stearic acid is written as 18 : 0, oleic acid, the only *cis* MUFA of major nutritional significance, as 18 : 1 and linoleic acid as 18 : 2.

The position of double bonds in a fatty acid is denoted by a numerical prefix, which is the number of the first carbon atom forming the double bond counting the carbon atom in the carboxyl group as number one (Figure 5.1). Linoleic acid is *cis*, *cis*-9,12-octadecadienoic acid and oleic acid is *cis*-9-octadecenoic acid.

Double bonds can also be numbered from the methyl group and this emphasizes relationships between different 'families' of fatty acids. Oleic acid is 18 : 1 (n-9), linoleic acid is 18 : 2 (n-6), γ-linolenic acid is 18 : 3 (n-6) and α-linolenic is 18 : 3 (n-3).

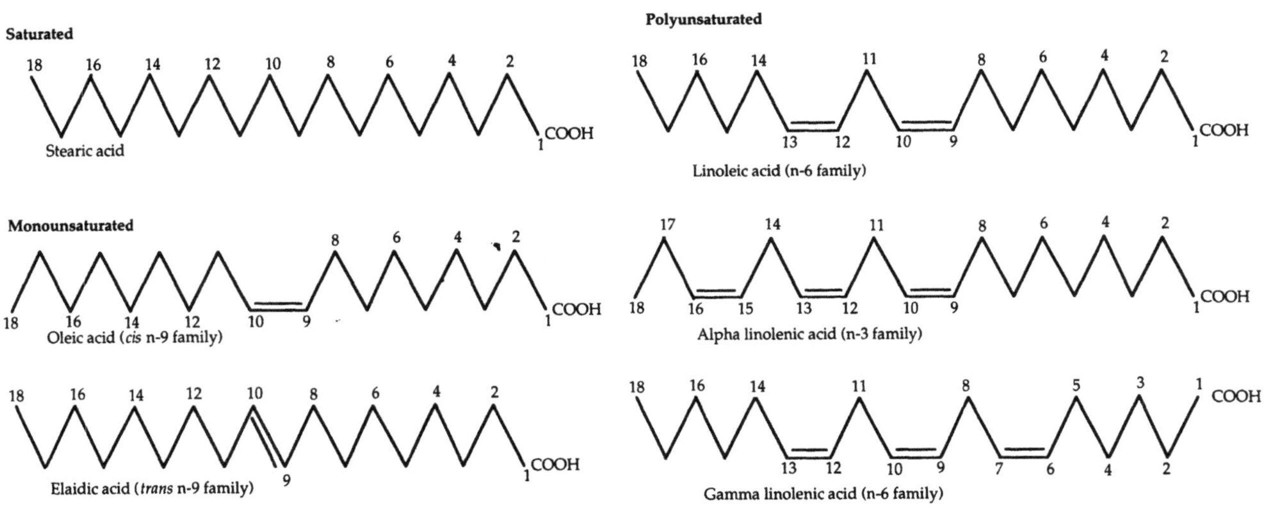

Figure 5.1 Chemistry of fatty acids. The carbon chains are represented by zig-zags with a carbon atom at each intersection. Double bonds are represented by double lines.

5.1.2 Characteristic fatty acids in different foods

All natural fats contain mixtures of SFA, MUFA and PUFA. Only the relative proportions change. What are loosely termed 'saturated fats' should more strictly be referred to as fats with a high proportion of SFA.

Ruminant fats (e.g. beef fat, butter) have a low proportion of PUFA because the PUFA in the animal's diet are hydrogenated by microorganisms in the rumen. Non-ruminants such as pigs and poultry tend to contain a higher proportion of PUFA in their storage fats depending on the nature of fatty acids in their feed.

Fish store fat either in the flesh (oil-rich fish such as herring and mackerel) or in the liver (cod). These fats are generally rich in long chain PUFA of the n-3 family such as eicosapentaenoic acid (EPA) (20 : 5 n-3) and docosahexaenoic acid (DHA) (22 : 6 n-3).

Storage fats of plants found in seeds and fruits vary widely in their fatty acid composition. Oleic acid (18 : 1) predominates in olive oil while linoleic acid (18 : 2 n-6) predominates in maize oil. Unusually for a plant oil, SFA rather than MUFA or PUFA, predominate in coconut oil.

Structural lipids generally contain a higher proportion of PUFA than most storage fats. The fat in beef muscle has more PUFA than beef storage fat. In animals, arachidonic acid (20 : 4 n-6) predominates, but in green leafy vegetables, α-linolenic acid (18 : 3 n-3) predominates.

5.1.3 Functions

Dietary fats are a concentrated source of energy, providing more than twice as many kilocalories (kcal) per gram as carbohydrates and protein. Triglycerides stored as adipose tissue function as an energy store. Fats also provide a source of the fat-soluble vitamins.

Dietary fats contain small amounts of phospholipids and cholesterol which have important functions in the body. Phospholipids are the main lipid component in the structure of biological membranes. They also stabilize the structure of lipoproteins, the particles which transport lipids in the blood.

Membrane phospholipids provide a store of PUFA that can be metabolized to molecules called eicosanoids that act as chemical messengers.

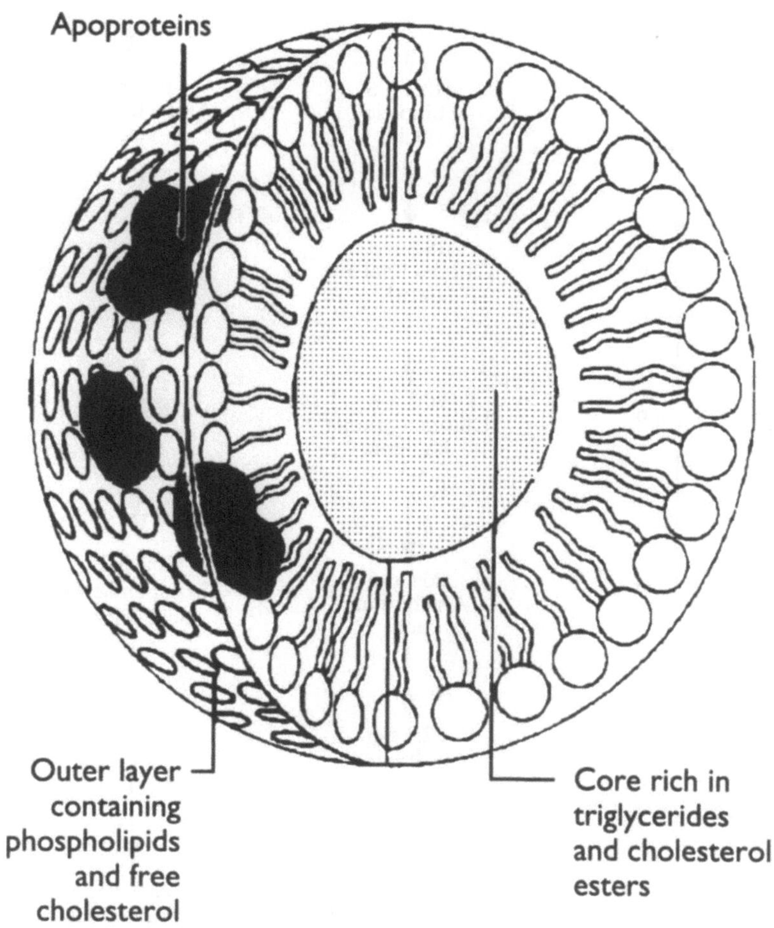

Figure 5.2 Diagram of a typical lipoprotein.

Specific phospholipids can also act as cell signalling devices.

Cholesterol is important for correct functioning of cell membranes. It acts as a precursor of steroid hormones, vitamin D, and bile acids which are involved in fat absorption. About three-quarters of the body's cholesterol is synthesized in body tissues and one-quarter comes from the diet.

5.1.4 Digestion, absorption and transport

Dietary fats are digested in the intestines to their component parts. After absorption the triglycerides are reassembled and transported in the blood as lipoproteins (see Figures 2.3 and 5.2). The protein component solubilizes the lipid and enables the particle to be 'recognized' by various tissues. This ensures lipid metabolism can be directed and controlled (Figure 5.2).

The liver can synthesize fats from carbohydrates and export them into the blood in the form of very low density lipoproteins (VLDL).

Diets in the UK contain sufficient fat so that the body does not usually need to make its own from carbohydrates. However, the liver can use spare fatty acids that circulate in the course of fat metabolism to make triglycerides and export them as VLDL.

Most of the cholesterol in the blood is carried by low density lipoproteins (LDL) which arise from the processing of VLDL. LDL transports cholesterol to tissues where it is required for the various functions listed earlier.

LDL particles have a protein on their surface called apoprotein B (apoB). This protein is 'recognized' by a receptor on the surface of the cells of various body tissues. It fits the receptor rather like a key fits into a lock. The LDL particles are then taken up into the cell where they deliver cholesterol

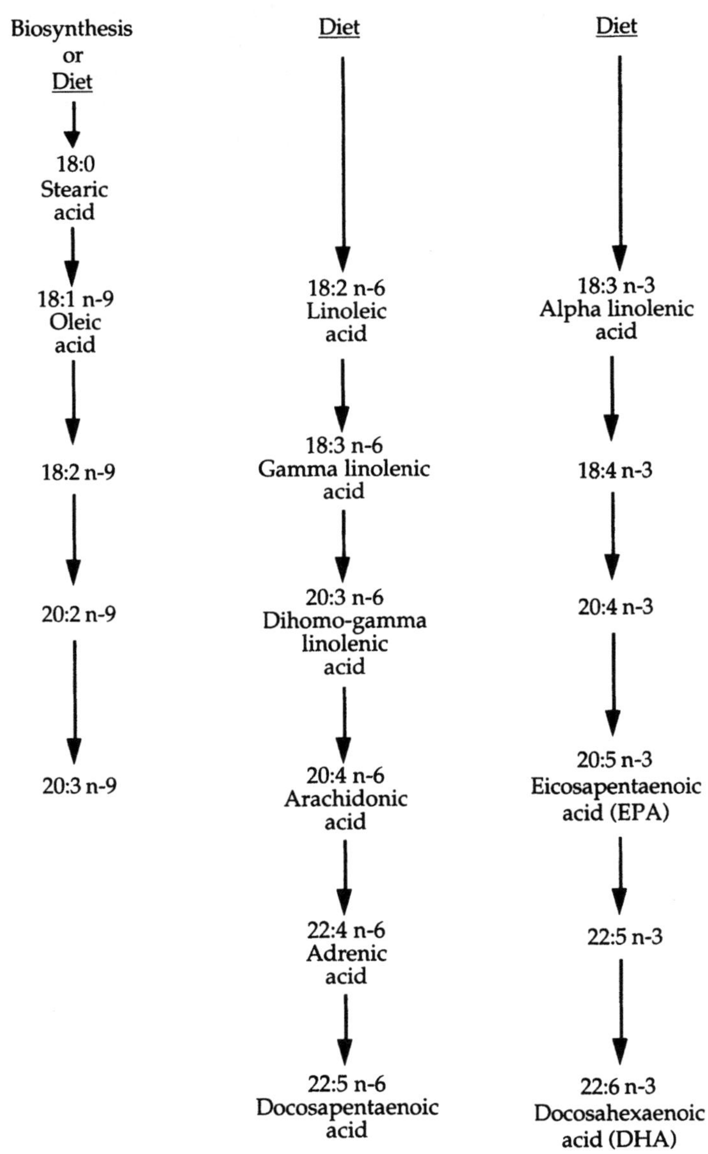

Figure 5.3 Metabolism of fatty acids.

and are able to regulate the cell's own capacity to synthesize cholesterol. The cells are able to make or destroy receptors continuously to comply with their demands for lipids.

Other particles, called high density lipoproteins (HDL) also carry cholesterol. They mainly retrieve it from places where too much has accumulated and carry it to the liver for disposal. Like other lipoproteins, HDL have a characteristic protein, in this case apoprotein A (apoA).

Sometimes LDL are altered chemically (e.g. by oxidation of the PUFA within them which then causes modification of the apoB). The oxidized particles are not recognized by the normal LDL receptors but are taken up by 'scavenger receptors' on blood cells called macrophages. Oxidized LDL particles are considered an important risk factor for CHD because they can have far-reaching effects on all stages of CHD (see Chapter 2).

5.1.5 Essential fatty acids

If required, the body can make SFA and MUFA itself, but most come from the diet. Two PUFA, linoleic acid (18 : 2 n-6) and α-linolenic acid (18 : 3 n-3) cannot be made in the body and are called essential fatty acids (EFA).

EFA can be incorporated into the body lipids or metabolized by the addition of more carbon atoms and more double bonds (Figure 5.3). These longer-chain, more highly unsaturated fatty acids are important components of cell membranes.

They can be converted into eicosanoids which have a variety of important biological activities. Eicosanoids influence smooth muscle contraction and blood clotting, mediate inflammatory reactions and regulate the immune system. The amounts and proportion of dietary fatty acids can influence the spectrum of eicosanoids and can have profound effects on the physiology of the body.

5.1.6 Dietary sources and intakes

The main sources of dietary fatty acids and cholesterol in the UK diet are shown in Table 5.1. Table 5.2 shows the content of total fat and individual fatty acids in a selected range of foods.

The major sources of SFA are milk and milk products such as cheese, meat and meat products such as pies and sausages, fat spreads (including butter and margarine), and cereal products such as biscuits and cakes. The average adult intake of SFA is about 16% of food energy (excluding *trans* fatty acids) (MAFF, 1995).

The major sources of *cis*-MUFA are meat, meat products, cereal products, milk and milk products, vegetables (including roast and fried) and fat spreads. The average adult intake of *cis*-MUFA is about 15% of food energy (MAFF, 1995).

The major sources of *trans* fatty acids are fat spreads (particularly hard margarine), meat and meat products and dairy products. The average adult intake is about 2% of total energy.

The major sources of n-6 PUFA are vegetables, cereal products, fat spreads and meat and meat products. The average adult intake of n-6 PUFA is about 7% of food energy.

The major dietary sources of n-3 PUFA are vegetables and vegetable oils, fat spreads, meat and meat products, and fish and fish products. The

Table 5.1 Major sources of dietary fatty acids and cholesterol in the UK diet (per person per day)

Food	SFA	*cis*-MUFA	*trans*-Fatty acids	n-6 PUFA	n-3 PUFA	Cholesterol
	g	g	g	g	g	mg
Milk and milk products	8.5	3.3	0.5	0.2	0.1	41
Fat spreads (including butter and margarine)	6.2	3.0	1.4	2.4	0.3	30
Meat and meat products	8.3	8.3	0.9	2.0	0.3	96
Fish and fish products	0.6	0.9	0.1	0.5	0.2	16
Eggs and egg dishes	1.1	1.4	0.1	0.5	0.0	154
Cereal products	6.6	4.7	1.3	2.6	0.3	19
Vegetables (including roast and fried)	2.4	3.2	0.3	2.8	0.4	10
Fruit and nuts	0.1	0.3	0.0	0.2	0.0	0
Sugar, confectionery and preserves	1.3	0.6	0.2	0.1	0.0	0
Beverages	0.2	0.0	0.0	0.0	0.0	0
Others	1.2	0.9	0.1	0.5	0.0	5
Total	36.5	26.7	4.8	11.7	1.6	371

From Gregory *et al.*, 1990 (except cholesterol, which is estimated).

Table 5.2 Sources of fat and fatty acids from 100g food

	Total fat g	SFA g	MUFA g	PUFA g
Avocado pear	19.5	4.1	12.1	2.2
Butter	81.7	54.0	19.8	2.6
Cheddar cheese	34.4	21.7	9.4	1.4
Coconut oil	99.9	85.2	6.6	1.7
Double cream	48.0	30.0	13.9	1.4
Eggs	10.8	3.1	4.7	1.2
Herring, grilled	8.8	3.7	5.9	2.1
Lard	99.0	40.8	43.8	9.6
Olive oil	99.9	14.0	69.7	11.2
Peanuts	46.1	8.2	21.1	14.3
Polyunsaturated margarine	81.7	16.2	20.6	41.1
Sardines, canned in tomato sauce	11.6	3.3	3.4	3.7
Sausage roll	36.4	13.4	15.6	5.3
Streaky bacon, grilled	36.0	14.1	16.3	3.8
Sunflowerseed oil	99.9	11.9	20.2	63.0
Whole milk	3.9	2.4	1.1	0.1

Source: Holland *et al.*, 1991.*

average adult intake of all n-3 PUFA is less than 1% of food energy. The major sources of the long chain n-3 PUFA (i.e. those with chains of 20 or 22 carbon atoms) are the oil-rich fish such as mackerel, herring and salmon. They contribute about 0.1% of total energy.

The major sources of dietary cholesterol are eggs and meat. The average adult intake of dietary cholesterol is 345 mg per person per day.

5.2 NON-STARCH POLYSACCHARIDES OR DIETARY FIBRE

5.2.1 Chemistry

Non-starch polysaccharides (NSP) (or dietary fibre) describe a mixture of substances present in plant cell walls and plant gums that are not digested in the small intestine (British Nutrition Foundation, 1990).

Plant cell wall materials in the diet include cellulose, hemicelluloses and pectic substances. Cellulose molecules are linear, unbranched polymers of glucose linked in β-1,4 geometry.

In contrast to the α-linkages of starch, this prevents cellulose from being digested by amylase.

The hemicelluloses consist of a mixture of polymers such as linear and branched xylose polymers with arabinose, glucose and glucuronic acid side chains. Pectic substances are a mixture of branched polymers with a galactose backbone and polymers of galacturonic acid.

Cellulose and hemicelluloses are insoluble in water, in contrast to pectic substances which are soluble. Plant gum materials, also soluble, are frequently used in food manufacture as thickeners and emulsifiers. These include locust bean gum, guar gum, alginates and carrageenan.

5.2.2 Fermentation

Bacteria present in the colon are able to ferment most forms of NSP, producing short-chain fatty acids which are absorbed into the blood stream. Apart from acting as useful metabolic precursors in various tissues, these acids influence the cells lining the large bowel and exert an effect on carbohydrate and lipid metabolism in the liver. They also have an important role in the control of salt and water levels in the colon.

Bacterial degradation of different forms of NSP is influenced by a number of factors including:

- the chemical structure of the fibre;
- its physical form; and
- the prevailing conditions within the colon.

Some forms of NSP are extensively degraded, notably those from vegetable and fruit sources, while others are more resistant, particularly that in bran.

5.2.3 Effect of NSP on absorption of sugars and fats

Soluble NSP retards absorption of glucose from the small intestine into the blood stream. This is believed to be due to production of viscous solutions near the wall of the small intestine, slowing diffusion of glucose and its precursors to the sites of absorption.

Some influence on fat absorption has also been observed following high doses of guar gum or pectin, leading to a reduction in plasma cholesterol concentration.

Animal experiments have suggested that NSP may modulate blood lipid levels. Soluble NSP such as oat bran and legumes can lower plasma cholesterol levels in human subjects. Other forms of soluble NSP such as guar gum have also been reported to lower plasma cholesterol concentration, while insoluble forms such as bran have inconsistent effects.

5.2.4 Dietary sources and intakes

Dietary intakes of total NSP among UK adults are around 12 g per day. Nearly half of NSP intake is from cereal products (mainly from bread), 38% from vegetables and 8% from fruit.

Absolute NSP intakes are higher in men, but intakes per 1000 kcal are slightly higher in women. About 45% of NSP consumed in the UK diet is in the soluble form. Table 5.3 shows the NSP content of a selected range of foods.

Table 5.3 Sources of starch and NSP from 100g food

	g Starch	g NSP
Baked beans in tomato sauce	9.4	3.7
Blackcurrants, stewed	0	3.6
Branflakes	50.6	13.0
Brown rice, boiled	31.6	0.8
Brussels sprouts, boiled	0.3	3.1
Lentils, red, boiled	16.2	1.9
Muesli	51.4	7.6
Peanuts	6.3	6.2
Peas, boiled	7.6	4.5
Raisins	0	2.0
Red kidney beans, boiled	14.5	6.7
White bread	46.7	1.5
Wholemeal bread	39.8	5.8
Wholewheat Spaghetti, boiled	21.9	3.5

Source: Holland *et al.*, 1991.*

5.3 STARCHES

5.3.1 Chemistry

Starches are polymers of the monosaccharide glucose. They vary in the number of glucose molecules they contain and in their arrangement. Starch granules are composed, in varying proportions, of a linear molecule amylose (200–300 glucose residues) and a branched molecule amylopectin (over 1000 glucose residues).

5.3.2 Digestion

The starches are digested by α-amylases and maltases which hydrolyse the glucosidic bond between the glucose residues. The resulting glucose molecules are absorbed in the small intestine and circulate in the blood causing a rise in blood glucose concentration.

This stimulates release of the hormone insulin, with blood insulin levels rising as blood glucose rises. Insulin release results in uptake of glucose from the blood by its action on a number of tissues including adipose tissue and muscle. The rate and extent of starch digestion is determined by:

- the properties of the starch granules;
- the effect of cooking and food processing;
- factors relating to the nearby structures in the food;
- extrinsic factors such as extent of chewing, transit time; and
- through the small intestine and the concentration of amylase.

The rate of starch digestion determines the rise in blood glucose and blood levels of insulin. This has important implications in metabolic disorders such as diabetes mellitus and CHD.

(a) Resistant starch

Some starch is not completely digested in the small intestine. Resistant starch (RS) passes into the large intestine where it is fermented by the colonic bacteria producing the short-chain fatty acids acetate, propionate and butyrate. Resistant starch may escape digestion in the small intestine for three reasons:

1. It is in a form which is physically difficult to get at, e.g. partly milled grains and seeds, or some very dense types of processed starchy food such as pasta; this type is called RS1.
2. It is in the form of particular starch granules which are highly resistant to digestion; this type is called RS2.
3. It has a large network of hydrogen bonds which stabilize the crystalline structure. This makes it particularly difficult for it to be hydrolysed by enzymes. This fraction is called RS3 and represents the extreme in resistance; it is mainly retrograded amylose.

RS1 and RS2 are the residues of starch forms which are partially digested in the small intestine.

RS3 is entirely resistant to digestion by pancreatic amylase. For many foods, RS1 and RS2 are quantitatively the most important types of resistant starch.

(b) Glycaemic index

Relative rates of absorption from different foods can be compared using the glycaemic index (GI) (Figure 5.4). Blood glucose levels are measured at regular intervals for 3 hours after eating a test food containing 50 g carbohydrate. The area under the curve is then compared with the one produced when the same subject eats 50 g carbohydrate from a standard source (glucose or white bread). If white bread is given a GI of 100, values range from less than 50 for legumes to 110 for mashed potato.

5.3.3 Effect on serum lipid levels

Excess glucose is converted in the liver to triglyceride and is stored in adipose tissue. In the short term, fasting levels of triglycerides rise on high carbohydrate diets, but return to normal in the long term. It has been suggested that high-carbohydrate diets may exacerbate any pre-existing insulin resistance.

5.3.4 Dietary sources and intakes

In general as the proportion of total energy from starch decreases the contribution from fat increases.

Carbohydrate typically provides just under half (45%) of total energy consumed (Gregory *et al.*, 1990). Just over half is consumed as starch. Mean daily intakes for men (156 g) are higher than for women although the difference is lost on adjustment for energy.

The main sources of starches in the UK are bread and flour, other cereal products such as rice and pasta, and potatoes. The average daily intake of starches provides approximately 520 kcal (2216 kJ). There is wide individual variation in intakes.

The major contributions to starch in the diet come from cereals (23% from bread alone), and vegetables where the largest single contribution is from potatoes. Table 5.3 shows the starch content of a selected range of foods.

5.4 ANTIOXIDANTS

The principal dietary antioxidant nutrients are vitamin C, vitamin E and carotene, of which fruits and vegetables are a main source. Other non-nutrient components in foods may have some degree of antioxidant activity, and many of these also occur in fruits and vegetables.

5.4.1 Vitamin C

Vitamin C (ascorbic acid) is considered the most important water-soluble antioxidant in extracellular

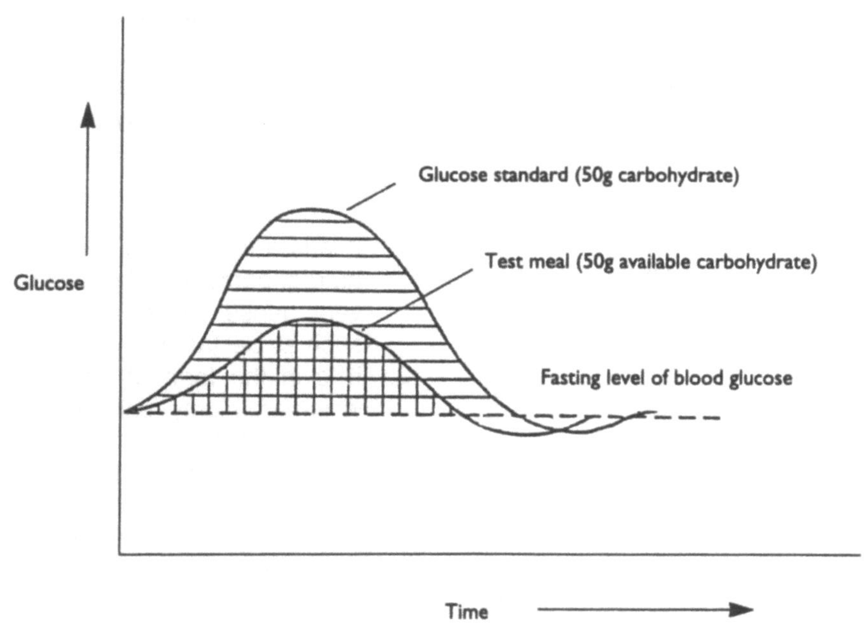

$$GI = \frac{\text{Area shaded in vertical bars} \times 100}{\text{Area shaded in horizontal bars}}$$

Figure 5.4 Determination of glycaemic index (GI). (Source: Jenkins *et al.*, 1981.)

fluids. The essential undisputed role of this vitamin involves hydroxylation reactions for the synthesis of collagen needed to prevent scurvy and aid wound healing. It also supports the absorption of non-haem iron, which may be especially important in those whose consumption of meat products is low.

5.4.2 Vitamin E

Vitamin E is the major lipid-soluble antioxidant in all cellular membranes and is the collective name for eight different tocopherols and tocotrienols. The most active compound, accounting for about 90% of the vitamin E in human tissue, is the RRR isomer of α-tocopherol.

Vitamin E deficiency states are rarely manifest in humans other than in premature infants where a specific syndrome comprising haemolytic anaemia may occur.

5.4.3 Carotenoids

Carotenoids are a group of pigments found mainly in plant foods, ranging in colour from yellow to dark red. While 500 naturally occurring carotenoids have been identified – many of which are biologically important antioxidants – only about 10% of these are able to serve as precursors of vitamin A.

β-Carotene has the highest vitamin A activity of any of the carotenoids, and is also one of the most widely distributed in nature; other carotenoids do not contribute significantly to vitamin A intakes in most normal diets.

For purposes of calculation, 6 μg of β-carotene are regarded as having the same vitamin A activity as 1 μg of retinol (retinol equivalents), while other pro-vitamin A carotenoids are ascribed the lower conversion factor of 12 : 1.

Other important carotenoids in the UK diet are lycopene (which is the major carotenoid of tomatoes) and lutein, which is found predominantly in green leafy vegetables.

5.4.4 Flavonoids

Flavonoids are a large group of polyphenolic antioxidants that occur naturally in vegetables and fruits and in beverages such as tea and wine. The most important groups of flavonoids are anthocyanins (such as malvidin and delphinidin), flavonols (such as kaempferol and quercetin), flavones (such as luteolin, rutin and apigenin), catechins (such as catechin and epicatechin), flavonones (such as naringen and taxifolin) and hydroxycinnamates (such as chlorogenic acid and caffeic acid).

5.4.5 Dietary sources and intakes

Table 5.4 shows the antioxidant nutrient content of a selected range of foods. The Dietary and Nutritional Survey of British adults (Gregory *et al.*, 1990) included an assessment of antioxidant nutrient intakes (Table 5.5).

Table 5.4 Sources of vitamins C, E and carotene from 100g food

	Vit C mg	Vit E mg	Carotene mg
Blackcurrants, stewed	115	0.8	0.1
Broccoli, boiled	44	(1.1)	0.5
Brussels sprouts, boiled	60	0.9	0.3
Carrots, boiled	2	0.6	7.6
Mangoes, raw	37	1.1	1.8
Plums, raw	4	0.6	0.3
Sweet potato, boiled	17	4.4	4.0
Tomatoes, raw	17	1.2	0.6

Source: Holland *et al.*, 1991.*

(a) Vitamin C

The average daily intake from foods was 67 mg for men and 62 mg for women. Inclusion of vitamin C from supplements increased average daily intakes to 75 mg and 73 mg respectively. Vegetables pro-

Table 5.5 Intake of antioxidant nutrients from food sources in UK adults 16 to 64 years

Antioxidant nutrient		Men	Women
Vitamin C	mg total intake	67	62
	mg per 1000 kcal/2185 kJ	28	38
Vitamin E	mg total intake	9.9	7.2
	mg per 1000 kcal/2185 kJ	4.1	4.3
Carotene	mg total intake	2.4	2.1
	mg per 1000 kcal/2185 kJ	1.0	1.3

Source: Gregory *et al.*, 1990.

vided nearly 50% of dietary vitamin C, with potatoes alone contributing 16%. Other major sources were fruit juice (18%) and fruit (17%). Intakes of vitamin C did not appear to be age-related although women consistently had higher intakes per unit energy than men.

(b) Vitamin E

The average daily intake from food sources was 9.9 mg for men and 7.2 mg for women. Vitamin E from supplements increased average intakes to 11.7 and 8.6 mg respectively.

Fats and oils provided almost half of the vitamin E, other important sources being green vegetables, nuts and eggs. Intakes of vitamin E did not vary with age in men, but were generally lower in young women. Unit energy intakes of vitamin E showed no significant sex differences or social class trends.

(c) Carotene and carotenoids

More than 80% of carotene consumed in the UK diet comes from vegetables, the largest single contribution coming from carrots. Small additional quantities of carotene come from yellow-fleshed fruits, fats and dairy products.

Intakes from food were 2.4 mg/day for men and 2.1 mg/day for women. In both sexes an increase with age was evident, indicating probably a more regular consumption of vegetables. Unit energy intakes for carotene showed higher intakes with increasing age, in subjects taking supplements, in subjects on slimming diets, and in social classes I and II compared with classes IV and V.

Average daily UK intake of lycopene is thought to be about 0.2 mg.

(d) Flavonoids

Daily intakes of the flavonoids quercetin, kaempferol, myrecetin, apigenin and luteolin have been estimated to be around 25 mg in the Netherlands (Hertog *et al.*, 1993). Intakes in UK are probably very similar.

5.5 SALT

5.5.1 Physiology

Salt, known chemically as sodium chloride, is composed of 40% sodium. When it dissolves in water it separates into its constituent ions, sodium and chloride, which are both vital constituents of body fluids and essential nutrients in the diet.

The body of a healthy 65-kg man contains approximately 92 g sodium, equivalent to 234 g of salt. About 50% of this is in the extracellular fluids, 40% in bone and 10% within the cells.

Sodium is essential for the maintenance of the correct blood volume and BP. It exerts a crucial effect on the passage of water into and out of the body's cells, and on the relative extracellular and intracellular fluid volume. The transmission of nerve impulses and contraction of the heart and other muscles are also dependent on sodium.

Sodium concentration in the body is maintained by several regulatory mechanisms and correlations between dietary sodium and urinary sodium excretion are weak.

5.5.2 Effect on blood pressure

High salt intakes have been associated with increased incidence of high BP but the relationship appears complex (see Chapter 6).

5.5.3 Dietary sources and intakes

Sodium in the diet tends to come less from sodium naturally present in foods, and more from salt added to foods during processing or the voluntary addition of salt to foods. The latter makes it difficult to assess sodium intakes accurately as practices between individuals vary widely.

The Dietary and Nutritional Survey of British Adults (Gregory *et al.*, 1990) assessed mean intakes of sodium, excluding discretionary salt, as 3.4 g/day for men and 2.4 g/day for women. These intakes are higher than physiological requirements.

From research examining total intakes of salt in the diet, using a marker to assess salt used in cooking and at the table, about 75% of dietary salt appears to come from salt added to foods during processing (Sanchez-Castillo *et al.*, 1987).

The National Food Survey (MAFF, 1994b) has estimated sodium content of the diet since 1985. It has never included salt in food eaten outside the home or discretionary salt. Values are therefore lower than those obtained from other surveys. The trend since 1986, however, shows a small decrease in average salt consumption from 6.7 g/day in 1986 to 6.3 g/day in 1992.

The National Food Survey also gives information on the sources of sodium in the household diet. For instance, the NFS showed that in 1992, bread provided about 17% of the sodium in foods brought into the home, meat products another 20%, while milk and dairy products such as cheese, fat spreads such as margarine, and vegetables including canned vegetables provided about 10% each. Breakfast cereals as a group only provided about 5% of sodium intakes.

The sodium content of a selected range of foods is shown in Table 5.6.

Table 5.6 Sources of sodium from 100g food

	mg Sodium
Baked beans in tomato sauce	530
Cheddar cheese	670
Fish cakes, fried	500
Prawns, shelled	1590
Salami	1850
Sausages, pork, grilled	1000
Smoked salmon	1880
Vegetable soup, canned	500
White bread	520

Source: Holland *et al.*, 1991.*

5.6 ALCOHOL

Ethyl alcohol (C_2H_5OH) is a dietary source of energy providing 7 kcal (29 kJ) per gram. Alcohol is unique in that it also has potent pharmacological effects. Unlike other dietary sources of energy, it cannot be metabolized by muscle directly, and is metabolized entirely in the liver at a fixed rate (0.1 g/kg body weight per hour). For example, a 55-kg woman would require $2\frac{1}{2}$ hours to metabolize the alcohol in a glass of wine.

The concentration of alcohol in beverages varies greatly (Table 5.7) but the volume consumed is usually a greater determinant of absolute alcohol intake. The new consensus advice issued by Government at the end of 1995 is that intake should not exceed 3 to 4 units a day for men and should not exceed 2 to 3 units a day for women (1 unit is 8 g or 10 ml alcohol). The recommendations were given as units per day rather than units per week to emphasize the point that it is 'binge' drinking which must be discouraged. The recommendations also stressed that the maximum health benefit was seen for middle-aged men and post-menopausal women. Sensible guidance on drinking levels for maximum health advantage lie in the recommendation of between 1 and 2 units a day for both sexes for these age groups only.

Table 5.7 Alcohol content of beverages

	Units of alcohol	**Alcohol g/100 ml**
Beer (284 ml)	1	2.6
Lager (284 ml)	1	3.2
Spirit (25 ml)	1	32
Cider (284 ml)	1.5	3.8
Wine (150 ml)	1.5	9.0

Source: Holland *et al.*, 1991.*
1 Unit is 8g or 10ml of alcohol.

The Dietary and Nutritional Survey of British Adults (Gregory *et al.*, 1990) recorded an average consumption of alcohol in men at 25.0 g/day, compared with 6.9 g/day for women. These figures include 21% of men and 35% of women who consumed no alcohol during the recording period. Alcohol intake among those who had consumed alcohol was considerably higher at 31.5 g/day for men and 10.6 g/day for women and was highest in the 25–49-year age range.

Men in the North tended to consume greater amounts of alcohol than men in the South East and London, and male alcohol consumers in social classes IV and V consumed more than males in other groups. These trends were not observed in women.

*Data from *The Composition of Foods*, 5th Edition are reproduced with the permission of The Royal Society of Chemistry and the Controller of Her Majesty's Stationery Office.

6

THE INFLUENCE OF DIETARY FACTORS ON DIFFERENT PHYSIOLOGICAL RISK FACTORS

(See the outer ring of the Round Table Model in the colour section)

6.1 INFLUENCE OF DIETARY FACTORS ON BLOOD PRESSURE (SEE FIGURE 6.1)

Systolic and diastolic BP are directly related to risk of CHD and stroke. The relationship appears to be linear, positive and continuous across a wide of range of pressures (Department of Health, 1994).

Increased BP is one of the physiological risk factors that can initiate or exacerbate arterial injury. The most important diet-related factors affecting BP are obesity, alcohol intake (particularly 'binge' drinking) and sodium intake. The ratio of sodium to potassium in the diet and the intake of fish oils rich in long-chain n-3 PUFA may also have an effect.

6.1.1 Obesity

Obesity is associated with increased BP (Department of Health, 1995b). On average, systolic BP is 0.8 mmHg higher for each unit increase in body mass index (BMI). An obese person with a BMI of 40 is likely to have a systolic BP about 16 mmHg higher than an average thin person with a BMI of 20, all other factors being equal.

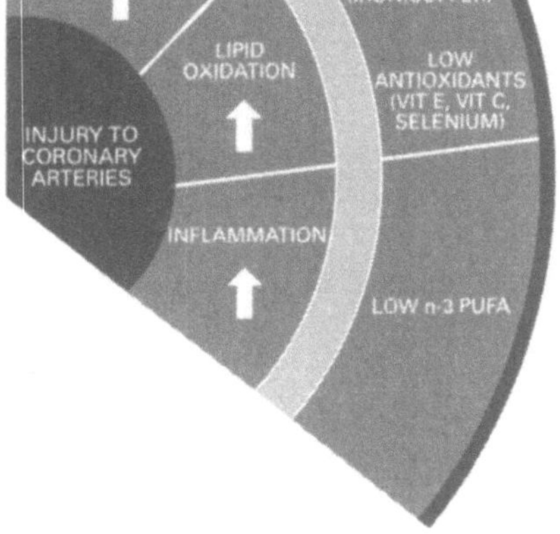

Figure 6.1 Dietary factors influencing physiological risk factors which lead to injury of the coronary arteries.

The relationship is especially strong when the excess fat is 'centrally' distributed around the trunk and abdomen because this indicates that the majority of the excess fat is located in the internal, visceral depots (Ashwell, 1996).

Of all the simple anthropometric indices which are proxies for central obesity, the ratio of waist circumference to height (WHTR) showed the closest association with blood pressure in a cross-sectional study of British adults (Lejeune *et al.*, in press).

6.1.2 Alcohol (particularly 'binge' drinking)

There have been many studies linking alcohol and increased BP over the last 20 years. Most studies show a dose-response relationship between drinking and diastolic and systolic BP, although about half the studies in women show a slight J-shaped relationship. A cautious interpretation of the evidence suggests that alcohol consumption results in a dose-dependent rise in BP with a possible plateau at about 80 g (10 units) a day.

A number of studies have shown that each increment of 10 g (1.25 units) of alcohol drunk per day increases systolic BP by an average of 1–2 mmHg and diastolic BP by 1 mmHg. A generally accepted clinical view is that for men the rise in BP produced by 4 units a day would give cause for concern. 'Binge' drinking is particularly associated with significantly raised BP and this is why the new guidelines on sensible drinking give recommendations on a daily, rather than a weekly, basis (Department of Health, 1995a).

Investigations into the mechanisms by which alcohol consumption affects BP usually conclude that alcohol is a vasodilator at low doses, but a pressor at higher doses (Victor and Hansen, 1995).

6.1.3 Sodium

Sodium is required for the maintenance of extracellular fluid volume and hence blood pressure (BP), and for the generation and transmission of electrical impulses in nerves and muscles and the uptake of certain nutrients from the small intestine. Based on physiological requirements, the Reference Nutrient Intake for sodium is 1.6 g/day (equivalent to 4.2 g salt/day) and the Lower Reference Nutrient Intake for sodium is 0.58 g/day (equivalent to 1.5 g salt/day) (Department of Health, 1991).

Two overviews of prospective studies and intervention trials of blood pressure and disease have found that reduction of BP has a much greater and more direct effect on reducing stroke rates than reducing coronary heart disease (CHD) risk (MacMahon *et al.* 1990; Collins *et al.*, 1990). This is probably because there are other risk factors for CHD and it is likely that the effects of prolonged elevated BP on CHD take longer to reverse than their effects on risk of stroke.

The effect of sodium intake on BP is usually deduced by looking at average salt intakes in different countries which have many cultural differences apart from diet. If this is done, there appears to be a strong relationship: BP is high if salt intake is high and low if salt intake is low. However, examining the intakes of individuals within countries does not show such a strong relationship (British Nutrition Foundation, 1994).

Two large surveys have been published which show that habitual sodium intake influences BP but have given somewhat different estimates of the magnitude of the relationship. The INTERSALT study was an inter-population comparison which estimated that the average systolic BP would rise by between 2–3 mmHg for every 100 mmol increase in daily sodium intake (equivalent to 6 g salt) (Intersalt Cooperative Research Group, 1988). A meta-analysis (Law *et al.*, 1991), estimated that systolic BP would, on average, rise by between 5–10 mmHg for every 100 mmol increase in sodium, depending on age.

Overall, the relationship between sodium intake and raised blood pressure is weak. Although there is good evidence that salt reduction can cause BP to fall – particularly in people with high BPs – there is disagreement among experts about whether this fall is enough to warrant a population reduction in salt intake. Some, but not others, believe that sodium intake can have a causal effect in raising BP, particularly the rise associated with increasing age. Some believe that other factors such as obesity and alcohol intake are more important (British Nutrition Foundation, 1994; Sadler *et al.*, 1995).

There is evidence that the ratio of sodium to potassium in the diet is more important than the absolute amount of either of these electrolytes in determining BP. The INTERSALT study showed that a 50% increase in potassium intake would result in an average reduction in systolic BP of 1.6 mmHg.

A World Health Organization (WHO) Technical Report (1990) proposed that population average salt intakes should not exceed 6 g per person per day and this recommendation was reiterated in The 1994 Coronary Review Group (COMA) (CRG) Report (Department of Health, 1994). This would require an average reduction of about one-third in salt intakes in the UK. It would be expected to have an impact on stroke rates, especially in the elderly, but a smaller effect on CHD rates in the short term. The magnitude of the effect is still debated (Swales, 1992) but the evidence is good enough to suggest that a reduction *together with* other proposed dietary changes and weight reduction in the overweight, could reduce BP and ultimately help to achieve the Health of the Nation CHD targets.

6.1.4 n-3 Polyunsaturated fatty acids

The long-chain n-3 PUFA, found almost exclusively in oil-rich fish, have been shown to reduce BP, particularly in people with high BP. Large intakes (5 g/day) of the n-3 fatty acids eicosapentaenoic acid (EPA) and docosahexaenoic acid (DHA) reduce BP by about 3–5 mmHg.

These amounts would be difficult to obtain from a normal 'Western' diet and would require the consumption of about 10 portions of oil-rich fish a week. The required amounts of EPA and DHA could only realistically be obtained from fish oil supplements.

It is possible that fish oil supplements can enhance the effect of salt restriction and that the combination of both measures is more effective for the reduction of BP than either acting alone.

6.2 INFLUENCE OF DIETARY FACTORS ON LIPID OXIDATION

6.2.1 Fatty acids

Theoretically, the LDL particles with a large proportion of unsaturated fatty acids are more prone to oxidation than those containing large proportions of saturated fatty acids (SFA) or *cis*-monounsaturated fatty acids (*cis*-MUFA). The benefits of increasing dietary PUFA therefore need to be balanced by potential disadvantages of increasing PUFA content of LDL particles.

MUFA, which lower LDL-cholesterol albeit to a lesser extent than PUFA, do not have the disadvantage of increasing LDL oxidizability. This is one reason why dietary guidelines usually set an upper limit on PUFA consumption but not on MUFA consumption.

For some unknown reason, increasing the amount of long-chain PUFA in the diet, with fish oil supplementation, does not appear to increase the oxidizability of LDL particles.

6.2.2 Pro-oxidants

Non-dietary factors such as smoking can promote oxidation but in relation to diet, attention is usually focused on copper and iron. Both are pro-oxidants and have the potential to catalyse the oxidation of LDL-cholesterol if they can exist in their free ionic form. However, they are normally prevented from initiating such damage because they are bound to transport proteins such as transferrin and ceruloplasmin.

The difference in iron status between men and women has been suggested as one explanation for the difference in CHD rates observed and has been put forward to explain the particularly low incidence in pre-menopausal women.

The concentrations of serum copper and serum ferritin (an index of iron stores), have been associated with increased risk of heart disease in one study. Men with plasma copper concentrations in the top third of the distribution were four times as likely to suffer a heart attack as men in the lowest third, while men with plasma ferritin levels above 200 μg/l were twice as likely to suffer a heart attack as those with levels less than 200 μg/l (Salonen *et al.*, 1992b).

Other studies have failed to show an association. For instance, 500 men (aged 35–54 years) did not show any difference in plasma iron or ferritin status in relation to their risk of angina (Riemersma *et al.*, 1991a).

In reviewing all the available evidence relating iron and CHD, the British Nutrition Foundation's Task Force concluded that the link between increased iron stores (as reflected by serum ferritin levels) and CHD risk is weak and the link between levels of dietary iron and CHD risk is even weaker. The increased serum ferritin levels found in some CHD patients are much more likely to reflect the role of ferritin as an acute phase marker rather than reflecting iron stores (British Nutrition Foundation, 1995b).

6.2.3 Antioxidants

Free radical attack can be reduced or prevented by antioxidants.

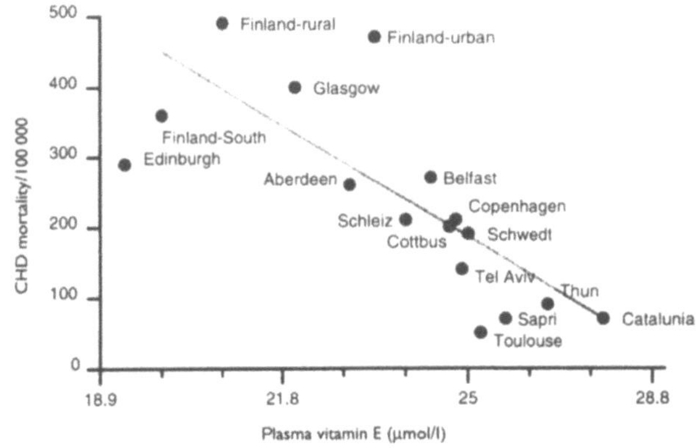

Figure 6.2 Plasma vitamin E and CHD mortality. (Source: Gey *et al.*, 1991.)

Several food components are able to act as antioxidants. Vitamin E, vitamin C and the carotenoids are usually regarded as the major dietary antioxidants. However, antioxidant activity can also be demonstrated in flavonoids found in fruits and vegetables, polyphenol fractions found in teas and phenolic substances found in red wines.

A cross-sectional survey of 16 000 men aged 40–59 years from 16 different European towns and cities found that concentrations of vitamin E in the blood were inversely related to death rates from CHD in the different populations (Figure 6.2) (Gey *et al.*, 1991). Populations with the lowest rates of CHD had the highest blood concentrations of vitamin E.

LDL is usually protected from oxidation by fat-soluble vitamin E contained within the lipoprotein. Vitamin E is able to break free radical chain reactions, preventing the damage from becoming too widespread. Vitamin E might be regenerated by the water-soluble vitamin C present in the plasma.

If the concentration of antioxidants is low, or if the LDL particle gets trapped in the artery wall so that vitamin E cannot be regenerated by plasma vitamin C, oxidation of PUFA molecules can overwhelm the antioxidant capacity of LDL and lead to oxidative modification of apoB.

Riemersma *et al.* (1991b) reported that the plasma concentration of vitamin E was inversely related to the risk of angina in a population case-control study in Scotland. The protective effect was strongest for vitamin E in subjects with the highest plasma vitamin E levels.

A previous study (Riemersma *et al.*, 1990) on plasma antioxidants and mortality from CHD in four European regions with differing CHD mortalities (North Karelia, eastern Finland; south-west Finland; Scotland; southern Italy) found that the differences in plasma antioxidants did not explain regional differences in CHD mortality although plasma vitamin E levels were lower in the high

CHD regions (Finland and Scotland in comparison with Italy).

Some of the variation in the CHD mortality seen across the different regions of Britain and some of the variation in social class differences can be explained by variations in levels of plasma antioxidants (MAFF, 1994a; Ashwell and Buss, 1995). Men and women in Scotland have lower levels than people in the South East and people in Social classes IV and V have lower levels than people in social classes I and II.

In two prospective studies on 40 000 men and 87 000 women in the USA (Rimm *et al.*, 1993; Stampfer *et al.*, 1993) a lower risk of CHD was observed in both groups for those taking high intakes of vitamin E as supplements for 2 or more years. A reduced risk was not observed for vitamin C supplements or dietary intakes of other antioxidant nutrients, other than a slight protective association for β-carotene in male smokers.

Recently, the results of several intervention trials have made some scientists question the ability of antioxidants to protect against cancer and CHD. The Alpha-Tocopherol, Beta-carotene Cancer prevention Study (ATBC) was a randomized, double-blind, placebo-controlled primary prevention trial to determine whether daily supplementation with 50 mg vitamin E, with 20 mg β-carotene, or with both, could reduce the risk of cancer in over 29 000 Finnish male smokers (Albanes *et al.*, 1994). The vitamin E-supplemented group showed no shifts in disease or death patterns. In contrast, the β-carotene-supplemented group had an 11% higher mortality rate from CHD, and although the increase was not as high as the increase in deaths from lung cancer (15%), the higher base-line incidence of CHD meant that the increase in absolute number of deaths was higher from this cause. Total mortality in the β-carotene group was increased by 8%.

In early 1996, the US National Cancer Institute announced that it was 'winding-up' the Beta-carotene and Retinol Efficacy Trial (CARET) because of an increase of 17% in all-cause mortality, an increase of 26% in death from cardiovascular causes and a 28% increase in morbidity from lung cancer among the 18 000 men considered to be at high risk of cancer because they had either been exposed to asbestos or they were smokers. The effects of β-carotene (30 mg) and vitamin A (25 000 IU) could not be distinguished because the two substances were given together (Omenn *et al.*, 1996).

The explanation put forward for these unexpected results was that both trials involved high-risk groups who were extra sensitive to the high levels of β-carotene used for supplementation.

Also in early 1996, the Physicians Health Study, which ended its nutritional intervention of 22 000 US male doctors at the end of the previous year, announced that β-carotene intervention (50 mg) had no effect on disease or death, even among the 'high-risk' smokers in this generally 'low risk' group (Hennekens *et al.*, 1996). This result was a relief to those worried about the possible harmful effects of β-carotene supplementation in healthy adults, but it was still a disappointment to those who had hoped to show positive effects from antioxidant supplementation. At the same time, the Iowa Women's study, which was a 7-year prospective study of 35 000 postmenopausal women, showed some benefit of vitamin E, but not vitamins A and C, from food in protecting against death from CHD (Kushi *et al.*, 1996).

The only intervention trial to produce some evidence of benefits from antioxidant supplementation has been the randomized controlled trial of vitamin E in patients with CHD known as the Cambridge Heart Antioxidant Study (CHAOS) (Stephens *et al.*, 1996). Over 2000 men and women were matched and assigned to vitamin E (either 800 IU or 533 mg daily for 2 years, reducing to 400 IU or 266 mg daily in half the patients) or to placebo treatment. Vitamin E reduced cardiovascular events and non-fatal myocardial infarctions (MI) quite dramatically, but there was a worrying increase in fatal MI and in total CVD deaths.

After the publication of the results of the ATBC trial, attention was focused on components of fruit and vegetables, apart from β-carotene. Other carotenoids and flavonoids were investigated to determine if it could be shown whether these compounds explain the protective properties of fruits and vegetables. Two epidemiological studies have provided some positive evidence for flavonoids.

In the Zutphen Elderly Study, Hertog *et al.* (1993) showed that older men with the highest intakes of flavonoids had the lowest risk of CHD 5 years later, even allowing for other possible confounding CHD risk factors.

In Finland, Knekt *et al.* (1996) related the usual diets of more than 5000 men and women to mortality from CHD 26 years later and showed protective effects for flavonoids, particularly those in apples and onions, indicating that quercetin was probably the flavonoid with the greatest protective properties.

Antioxidants may protect against free-radical initiated damage and protect LDL-cholesterol from oxidation. Since oxidized LDL-cholesterol is thought to be involved in the initial arterial injury and the formation of the fibrous plaque (see Chapter 2), protection by antioxidants has great potential in the prevention of CHD.

The recent evidence would indicate that it will not be as easy to identify specific antioxidant nutrients with 'magic bullet' properties as might have been thought a few years ago. The combination and interaction of a range of compounds with antioxidant function as they would naturally occur in a range of fruits and vegetables is obviously necessary for protection.

6.3 INFLUENCE OF DIETARY FACTORS ON INFLAMMATION

6.3.1 n-3 Polyunsaturated fatty acids

The cell types involved in inflammation include lymphocytes, macrophages, leukocytes and non-specific killer cells. The cell membranes all contain phospholipids which can be broken down to release free fatty acids.

Arachidonic acid and EPA are released readily and give rise to inflammatory eicosanoids: the prostaglandins and the leukotrienes. Figure 6.3 shows that the eicosanoids produced from arachidonic acid are more inflammatory than those produced by EPA. Dietary supplementation with oil-rich fish or EPA can distort the balance of fatty acids within the membrane phospholipids and help to reduce the inflammatory response.

6.4 INFLUENCE OF DIETARY FACTORS ON THE ATHEROGENIC LIPID PROFILE (SEE FIGURE 6.4)

The fibrous plaque grows by the combination of lipid deposition, the incorporation of small thrombi and the multiplication of smooth muscle cells (see Chapter 2).

Certain physiological conditions favour progression of the initial arterial injury into developed atherosclerotic lesions (see Chapter 3) but the process takes place over decades. Dietary factors and other behavioural factors, such as exercise, which influence these physiological conditions, moderate the rate of progression and development of the atherosclerotic lesions.

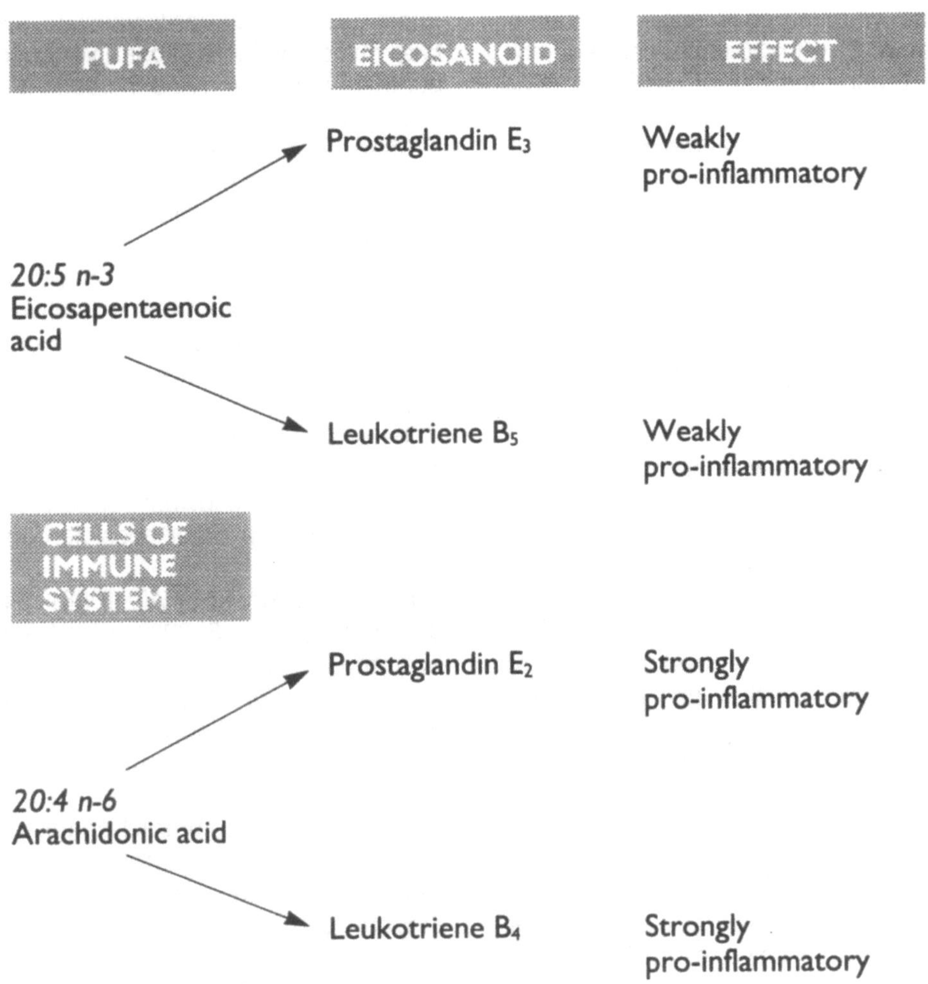

Figure 6.3 Formation of eicosanoids from n-3 and n-6 PUFA; their effects on inflammation.

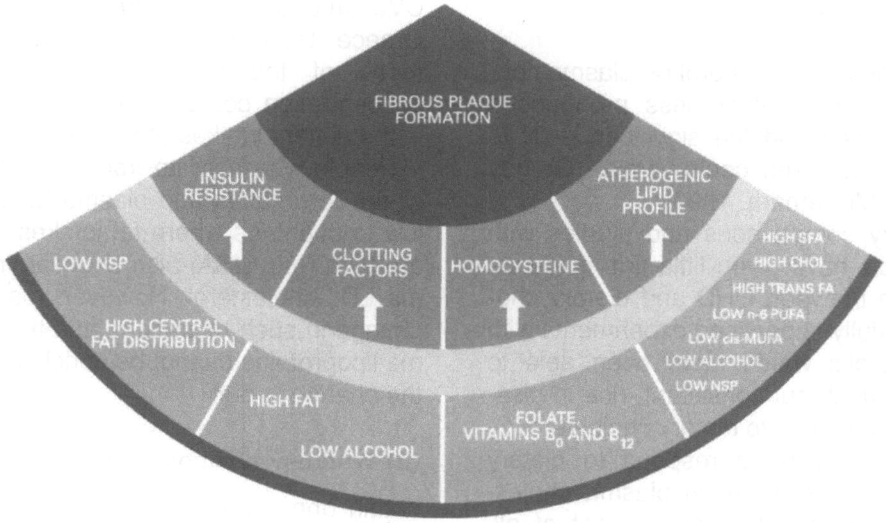

Figure 6.4 Dietary factors influencing physiological risk factors which lead to fibrous plaque formation.

6.4.1 Dietary lipids in general

Middle-aged men with high levels of plasma cholesterol >7.2 mmol/l have $3\frac{1}{2}$ times the risk of a heart attack than men with levels <5.5 mmol/l. In particular, high levels of LDL-cholesterol and low levels of high density lipoprotein (HDL) cholesterol are associated with increased risk of lipid deposition in the fibrous plaque and of CHD (see Chapter 3). The association between elevated plasma cholesterol and increased risk of CHD appears less consistent in women (Jacobs *et al.*, 1992).

Studies have found that plasma lipoprotein fractions can be altered in a predictable way by substituting one type of dietary fat for another. The main dietary fats found to influence plasma lipids were SFA, PUFA and cholesterol. The combined effects were originally summarized by Keys in the relationship:

$$\Delta\text{plasma cholesterol} = 2.7\,\Delta\text{SFA} - 1.35\,\Delta\text{PUFA} + 1.5\,\Delta\text{C}$$

where Δplasma cholesterol is the average change in the concentration of total plasma cholesterol in a group of people resulting from changes in intakes of SFA (ΔSFA) and in PUFA (ΔPUFA) expressed as percentages of energy provided by these lipids (mainly in the form of triglycerides) and the change in dietary cholesterol (ΔC) expressed as mg cholesterol per 1000 kcal, 4184 kJ.

Hegsted *et al.* (1993) have now refined this equation as follows:

$$\Delta\text{plasma cholesterol} = 1.35\,(2\,\Delta\text{SFA} - \Delta\text{PUFA}) + 1.5\,(\Delta\text{Z})$$

where ΔZ = the difference between the square roots of dietary cholesterol in the diets.

This new equation gives less emphasis to the effects of dietary cholesterol than the original equation but still emphasizes that the ability of SFA to raise plasma cholesterol is double the ability of PUFA to lower it.

These equations are still widely used to predict the response in plasma cholesterol if the intake of dietary fat is changed. Although they can give remarkably close predictions, they can be unreliable on some occasions for two reasons:

1. They do not take account of the fact that different types of PUFA and SFA have widely different effects on plasma cholesterol.
2. They do not include a term for MUFA which in earlier studies were found to be neutral in their effects but sometimes appear to lower plasma cholesterol levels when substituted for SFA.

Much of the experimental work is difficult to interpret because:

- of the impossibility of changing only one variable at a time;
- dietary interactions may result in different effects with practical mixed diets than when 'pure' fats and oils are used as supplements; and
- natural oils also contain minor components in addition to triglycerides which are different in each oil and may influence lipoprotein metabolism in unknown ways; e.g. corn or maize oil contains a large proportion of tocopherols, especially γ-tocopherols, and maize and palm oils contain tocotrienols that inhibit a key enzyme in cholesterol synthesis.

6.4.2 Dietary cholesterol

The influence of dietary cholesterol on plasma concentration in humans is much less pronounced than in other primates and the significance of its influence has always been controversial (Grundy and Denke, 1990; McNamara, 1990).

Between-country comparisons and studies with 'free-living' subjects have given little firm evidence for an association between CHD and dietary cholesterol. Only carefully supervised experiments with subjects in metabolic wards have been able to demonstrate the small, but consistent, rise in plasma cholesterol in response to dietary cholesterol.

Some individuals seem to respond to dietary cholesterol with a marked rise in plasma cholesterol, while others respond weakly or not at all. High intakes of dietary cholesterol may suppress LDL receptor activity in responsive subjects, enhancing the potential of certain SFA to raise cholesterol levels.

On the other hand, the greatest change in plasma cholesterol can be observed when dietary cholesterol is added to diets where baseline dietary cholesterol intakes are low (<100 mg/day). Little change is observed if baseline dietary cholesterol intakes are high (500 mg/day) (Hopkins, 1992).

Hegsted *et al.* (1993) produced an overview of the effects of dietary cholesterol on plasma cholesterol and concluded that 'dietary cholesterol increases plasma cholesterol and must be considered when the effects of fatty acids are evaluated' (see section 6.4.1).

The 1994 CRG Report (Department of Health, 1994) concluded that 'The weight of evidence supports the view that raising cholesterol levels in the diet increased plasma cholesterol, primarily LDL-cholesterol, although there is considerable variation in inter-individual response'. The Report also raised the possibility that dietary cholesterol may influence CHD risk by a mechanism other than through plasma cholesterol.

6.4.3 Saturated fatty acids

(a) Cross-community comparisons

Countries in which people have a high average SFA intake expressed as a percentage of energy, tend to have high rates of CHD, and national average SFA supplies correlate closely with national average plasma cholesterol levels (Shaper, 1988).

Both national and international studies demonstrate a strong association between intakes of SFA expressed as a percentage of dietary energy and CHD mortality (Keys, 1970). In Keys' Seven Countries Study, a study of diet and risk factors for CVD among healthy volunteers in Holland, Japan, Greece, USA, Yugoslavia, Finland and Italy, two-thirds of the variation in plasma cholesterol concentration could be predicted from differences in the dietary intakes of SFA and cholesterol.

People who migrate from countries (e.g. Japan) where fat intakes and plasma LDL-cholesterol are low to countries where fat intakes, especially SFA, are high (e.g. USA) also show an increase in plasma LDL-cholesterol. However, many other factors change in such migrations and the change in plasma lipoproteins cannot be conclusively attributed to the change in diet.

(b) Within-population studies

Within one country, people who die from CHD or have higher LDL-cholesterol levels do not generally eat more SFA or less MUFA and PUFA than those who do not die from CHD.

The difficulty in demonstrating a consistent association between fatty acid intakes and plasma cholesterol within a population is, in part, because there is often little variation in fatty acid intakes between individuals in a population and wide variation in any one individual. This tends to obscure any relationship that might exist.

Most of the variance in plasma cholesterol levels within a population reflects genetic variance. However, if groups with widely varying fatty acid intakes are compared then a significant relationship between SFA intake and plasma cholesterol can be seen.

Comparisons between strict vegetarians and meat-eaters show marked differences in plasma cholesterol levels that can be explained almost entirely by differences in SFA intakes (Sanders and Roshanai, 1984). Similar comparisons have been made between farmers from different parts of France who have different fat intakes (Renaud *et al.*, 1986).

Studies using dietary survey methods for the assessment of dietary intakes have a number of drawbacks. One study which measured the fatty acid composition of adipose tissue (an indicator of the proportions but not the amounts of the fatty acids consumed habitually) found this and, presumably, the fatty acid composition of the diet explained only a small percentage of the variation in plasma lipids in people with normal plasma lipid concentrations (Berry *et al.*, 1986).

The Dietary and Nutritional Survey of British Adults in over 2000 men and women (Gregory *et al.*, 1990) found that SFA intake as a percentage of food energy was positively associated with total plasma cholesterol in men and women, and with HDL and LDL-cholesterol in women, but not in men.

A study in 653 middle-aged men in Caerphilly also found a small positive association between the intake of SFA and LDL-cholesterol. However, diet as a whole accounted for less than 10% of the variation in plasma LDL and HDL concentrations and less than 2% in total plasma cholesterol (Fehily *et al.*, 1988).

(c) Prospective studies

Prospective studies have generally demonstrated a positive relationship between total plasma cholesterol concentrations and subsequent CHD but have been less consistent in their findings on fat consumption and subsequent CHD. The follow-up to the Seven Countries Study is the only international prospective study of diet and CHD. This found higher SFA intakes in people who went on to have heart attacks than in people who did not (Keys, 1980).

Other prospective studies have been carried out in single populations and have been reviewed recently (British Nutrition Foundation, 1992c). Two out of six studies found higher SFA intakes in people who subsequently had a heart attack compared with people who did not. However, four out of the six studies found that people who had heart attacks had lower or similar SFA intakes, expressed as a percentage of energy.

Four out of seven prospective studies found the ratio of PUFA to SFA (P/S ratio) was lower in those people who subsequently developed CHD than in those who did not, two found the P/S ratio was higher and one found it was identical (British Nutrition Foundation, 1992c). In a study in the USA, the correlation between the P/S ratio and plasma lipid concentration was small (Shekelle *et al.*, 1981).

(d) Intervention studies

Five large primary prevention trials on risk of CHD and death from all causes have suggested that advice to partly replace SFA by n-6 PUFA reduces the risk of a CHD event, but it has not been shown to reduce the risk of death (British Nutrition Foundation, 1992c).

The number of subjects in the trials ranged from 846 men to 60 881 men and the follow-up period ranged from 6 to 10 years. The trials were multifactorial; the intervention package included advice about other CHD risk factors such as smoking as well as advice on diet.

Four large intervention studies used dietary manipulation to lower blood cholesterol level – the Los Angeles Veterans Study (Dayton *et al.*, 1969), the Minnesota Coronary Survey (Frantz *et al.*, 1989), The Finnish Mental Hospitals Study (Turpeinen *et al.*, 1979), and the Oslo Study (Hjermann *et al.*, 1981). All resulted in a reduction of plasma cholesterol by about 13 to 16% from initial values.

These trials involved stringent diets with populations with high initial plasma cholesterol levels. Diets followed by free-living subjects rarely lower plasma cholesterol by more than 1 to 2% (Ramsay *et al.*, 1991).

Secondary prevention trials have also failed to demonstrate a convincing reduction in deaths from CHD and total deaths by the partial replacement of SFA by n-6 PUFA. There have been five randomized control trials of middle-aged men with the number of subjects ranging from 80 to 2033 and the length of follow-up period ranging from 2 to 11 years.

In these trials, the P/S ratio of diets for people in the intervention group ranged from 1.0 to 2.6. Because of the small sample sizes, most of these studies had a low probability of detecting any beneficial effect (British Nutrition Foundation, 1992c).

(e) Individual saturated fatty acids

Not all SFA are equivalent in their potential to raise plasma cholesterol levels (Ulbricht and Southgate, 1991).

Fatty acids with chain lengths up to and including 10 carbon atoms (short- and medium-chain fatty acids) have not been shown to influence plasma cholesterol because they are absorbed directly into the blood and rapidly metabolized in the liver.

Stearic acid (18 : 0) does not affect LDL-cholesterol, possibly because it is rapidly metabolized to oleic acid (18 : 1). Lauric (12 : 0), myristic (14 : 0) and palmitic (16 : 0) acids were originally regarded as the three 'cholesterol-raising' fatty acids affecting total and LDL-cholesterol concentrations. Myristic acid is probably the most potent and has been estimated to have four times the effect of the other two SFA. Palmitic acid is the principal SFA in most diets. There is now some evidence to suggest that it may not raise plasma cholesterol as much as myristic acid, provided that intakes of n-6 PUFA (linoleic acid) are above a certain threshold and intakes of dietary cholesterol are low (Hayes and Khosla, 1992).

The importance of SFA as a group being responsible for 'cholesterol-raising' effects of diets may have to be re-evaluated. It is possible that SFA intakes are only important in those people consuming significant quantities of full-fat dairy products, foods containing coconut and palm kernel oils (the major sources of lauric and myristic acids), and low levels of n-6 PUFA.

Despite much research, the mechanism by which specific SFAs raise LDL-cholesterol is not fully understood. Plausible explanations for why certain SFAs raise LDL levels include:

- inhibiting removal of LDL from plasma by interfering with LDL receptors in the liver; and
- stimulating LDL synthesis directly.

Apart from different responses to different SFAs, individuals have been shown to differ in their sensitivity to changes in cholesterol induced by dietary SFA reduction presumably reflecting an interaction between polygenic and other factors. Initial cholesterol and TG levels, apoB, apoE4 allele and CETP activity were all suggested as discriminating factors which could identify people who responded to a reduced SFA intake with the greatest decrease in plasma cholesterol (Cox *et al.*, 1995).

6.4.4 *cis*-Monounsaturated fatty acids

The only *cis*-MUFA of nutritional significance is oleic acid (18 : 1 n-9), but it normally makes the greatest single contribution of all fatty acids to the diet and is also the single most important fatty acid in the body in quantitative terms.

In early experiments *cis*-MUFA were thought to be 'neutral' in their effect on plasma cholesterol and did not figure in the Keys summary equation. Recent studies then found that when substituted for SFA, *cis*-MUFA lowered plasma cholesterol concentration almost as effectively as n-6 PUFA. The reduction was mostly in LDL-cholesterol. When substituted for carbohydrates, *cis*-MUFA resulted in a similarly low plasma LDL-cholesterol but did not elicit the rise in VLDL (and therefore triglycerides) often seen with high carbohydrate diets. Neither did they lower HDL-cholesterol. An overview of the effect of *cis*-MUFA by regression analysis showed no evidence of an independent effect of *cis*-MUFA on plasma cholesterol (Hegsted *et al.*, 1993).

In studies relating *cis*-MUFA intakes to CHD, four out of six investigations found higher MUFA intakes in people who subsequently had a heart attack compared with people who did not. It is possible then that any 'protective effect' of MUFA might result from effects other than an effect on lowering LDL-cholesterol.

The 1994 CRG Report concluded that substitution of SFA in the diet with oleic acid, a monounsaturated fatty acid, lowers both total and LDL-cholesterol in the plasma (Department of Health, 1994).

cis-MUFA are less susceptible to oxidation than PUFA and foods containing them may have a longer shelf-life. There is also some evidence that LDL-cholesterol particles containing a high proportion of oleic acid compared with linoleic acid are less susceptible to oxidation. Since oxidized LDL is now thought to be more important than native (not oxidized) LDL in the development of atherosclerosis (see Chapter 2); this could partly explain some of the beneficial effects of MUFA.

6.4.5 *trans* fatty acids

The effects of *trans* fatty acids on plasma cholesterol have been reviewed a number of times with conflicting conclusions (British Nutrition Foundation, 1987, 1995a).

High *trans* fatty acid intakes (10% of dietary energy, compared with current average UK intakes of 2% dietary energy) have been shown to raise LDL-cholesterol and to lower HDL-cholesterol (Mensink and Katan, 1990).

Data from a prospective study on over 80 000 women considered *trans* fatty acid intake calculated from dietary questionnaires. After adjustment for age and total energy intake, a positive relationship was found between *trans* fatty acid intakes and the risk of CHD (highest intakes 1.5 times lowest intakes) (Willett *et al.*, 1993).

The British Nutrition Foundation's most recent Task Force Report on *trans* Fatty Acids (1995a) concluded that:

> '*trans* fatty acids are qualitatively different to saturated fatty acids in their effects on HDL-cholesterol – saturated fatty acids raise HDL-cholesterol while *trans* fatty acids lower it. *trans* fatty acids raise LDL-cholesterol to approximately the same extent as saturated fatty acids. There is convincing evidence that *trans* fatty acids have an adverse effect on plasma LDL and HDL-cholesterol concentrations and this would appear to be greater than the adverse effect of an equivalent amount of saturated fatty acids'.

The most consistent evidence for the effect of a dietary component on Lp(a) levels is the effect of *trans* fatty acids. Several groups have shown that a diet high in *trans* fatty acids increased Lp(a) levels, by about 30% in some cases. (British Nutrition Foundation, 1995a).

6.4.6 Polyunsaturated fatty acids

(a) n-6 PUFA

The major effect of substituting n-6 PUFA for SFA, is a reduction of plasma cholesterol, principally the LDL fraction. There is little reduction in HDL-cholesterol as long as the contribution of linoleic acid is not more than 12% of dietary energy. This level is unlikely to be exceeded in most self-selected diets in the UK.

Plausible explanations for why unsaturated fatty acids, such as oleic and linoleic acids might lower LDL include:

- over-riding the inhibition in LDL receptor activity caused by certain SFA;
- lowering LDL-cholesterol by counteracting the increase in LDL synthesis caused by certain SFA; and
- simply substituting for SFA which raise LDL levels.

Only two out of six prospective studies found lower PUFA intakes in people who went on to have a heart attack (British Nutrition Foundation, 1992d).

A recent study has compared the fatty acids in serum and adipose tissue with the fatty acid composition of aortic plaques and shown a direct influence of dietary polyunsaturated fatty acids, but not saturated fatty acids on aortic plaque formation (Felton *et al.*, 1994). The authors suggested that the protective effects of increased intakes of polyunsaturated fatty acids towards CHD may have been overstated.

(b) n-3 PUFA

In contrast to n-6 PUFA, the main effect of n-3 PUFA is to reduce the concentration of VLDL. Since the major lipid component of these lipoproteins is triglyceride, the main response is lowering of plasma triglyceride concentrations. Only at very high intakes does n-3 PUFA lower LDL or total cholesterol.

The dramatic effect of a Mediterranean α-linolenic acid-rich diet in the secondary prevention of CHD (70% reduction in coronary events and cardiac events) was achieved without reduction in serum cholesterol, TG or an increase in HDL-cholesterol compared with controls (de Lorgeril *et al.*, 1994). The effect might have been due to an effect on reducing the risk of thrombosis (see section 6.10.2).

(c) Postprandial lipaemia

The effects of dietary fatty acid composition on the magnitude of postprandial lipaemia have only recently been reported. The findings show that as far as long-chain fatty acids are concerned, the magnitude of postprandial lipaemia decreases with increasing unsaturation (Table 6.1; see also Figure 3.2).

Unsaturated fatty acids of the n-3 series seem to have the most pronounced beneficial effect on postprandial TG. Fatty acids of the n-6 series also decrease postprandial TG levels but to a lesser extent than n-3 PUFA. In acute meal studies, substitution of SFA with MUFA has little effect on postprandial lipaemia (Zampelas, 1994). However, Greek subjects who are habituated to a high MUFA diet show less pronounced postprandial lipaemia than UK subjects after the same meal (Williams *et al.*, 1995).

In future, greater emphasis will probably be placed on the need to maintain low fasting and postprandial TG responses. Changes in the diet, including increased consumption of foods rich in n-3 PUFA as well as increased physical activity, appear to be the most effective means of achieving this goal.

6.4.7 Soluble non-starch polysaccharides

People who eat large amounts of NSP are less likely to die from CHD than those who eat smaller amounts. Different studies have found cereal fibre or vegetable fibre to be the most protective (British Nutrition Foundation, 1990).

An intervention trial in people who had already had one heart attack found that increasing the amount of cereal fibre in the diet had no effect on reducing CHD deaths during the following 2 years. Cereal fibre, especially from wheat, contains mainly insoluble NSP.

Table 6.1 Effect of different fatty acids on postprandial lipaemia (From Zampelas, 1994)

Long-chain saturated fatty acids	Increased postprandial TG responses, especially if background diet rich in saturated fatty acids.
Polyunsaturated fatty acids (n-6)	Slightly decreased postprandial TG responses, especially if background diet rich in polyunsaturated fatty acids (n-6)
Monounsaturated fatty acids (n-9)	Neutral effect on postprandial TG responses
Polyunsaturated fatty acids (n-3)	Large decrease in postprandial TG responses

More recent evidence suggests that it is the soluble NSP characteristically found in oats, vegetables and legumes, which are effective at lowering plasma LDL-cholesterol. Although addition to the diet of soluble NSP, such as those found in guar gum, oats and beans, reduces plasma cholesterol levels, there is some doubt whether these effects demonstrated over the short term, can be sustained in the long term.

Oat bran may selectively lower LDL-cholesterol, leading to a more favourable LDL/HDL-cholesterol ratio. An analysis of 19 trials found that oat bran or oatmeal both have a modest effect on reducing plasma cholesterol depending on the amount of soluble NSP and the initial plasma cholesterol (Ripsin *et al.*, 1992). The average reduction in total cholesterol was 0.13 mmol/l. Larger reductions (0.41 mmol/l) were seen in people with plasma cholesterol levels >5.9 mmol/l.

Table 6.2 shows how the reduction in cholesterol varied with the amount of soluble NSP and initial cholesterol levels; 3 g of soluble NSP is equivalent to one large bowl of ready-to-eat oat bran cereal.

A number of suggestions have been put forward for the mechanism by which soluble NSP can reduce plasma cholesterol:

1. Soluble NSP may bind to cholesterol and bile acids (derived from cholesterol) in the small intestine preventing re-absorption. The bound cholesterol would be excreted and the overall effect of this 'cholesterol drain' would be to decrease the amount of cholesterol in the circulation.
2. Soluble NSP are fermented by the colonic bacteria. One of the end-products is the short-chain fatty acid, propionate. This is known to inhibit cholesterol synthesis in the liver but it is uncertain whether the small amounts of propionate produced would have a significant effect.
3. Soluble NSP help to slow the absorption of glucose in the small intestine, resulting in lower concentrations of blood insulin. This may decrease cholesterol synthesis at least in the short term.

6.4.8 Starches

The fraction of starch not digested in the small intestine – resistant starch – is fermented in the colon and behaves very much like NSP. Theoretically, diets containing large amounts of resistant starch might reduce plasma cholesterol, but no experimental evidence is available.

6.4.9 Alcohol

Alcohol can influence lipid metabolism and several studies have demonstrated a positive association between alcohol consumption and increased plasma HDL-cholesterol (Castelli *et al.*, 1977; Linn *et al.*, 1989). In addition, alcohol lowers LDL-cholesterol levels (Department of Health, 1995a) and it is thought to be through these lipoprotein cholesterol pathways that alcohol inhibits the formation of the fibrous plaque. In fact, the inverse association between alcohol consumption and risk of CHD in men has been shown to be highly dependent on the concentration of LDL-cholesterol (Hein *et al.*, 1996).

Among women, light to moderate alcohol consumption has also been associated with a reduced mortality rate, but this apparent survival benefit appears largely confined to post-menopausal women (Fuchs *et al.*, 1995).

Phenolic substances in red wine have been shown to inhibit oxidation of human LDL in vitro (Frankel *et al.*, 1993). All of these mechanisms may help to explain the 'French paradox' (the lower than expected incidence of CHD in France in relation to SFA intake).

A recent review of 25 different studies in men and women relating moderate alcohol consumption to the reduced risk of CHD concluded that all alcoholic drinks are linked with lower risk, thus implying

Table 6.2 The reduction in plasma cholesterol (mmol/l) achieved according to the amount of soluble NSP and initial cholesterol levels

Amount of soluble NSP	**Reduction in plasma cholesterol level (mmol/l)**	
	Initial plasma cholesterol <5.9 mmol/l	**Initial plasma cholesterol >5.9 mmol/l**
<3 g/day	0.09	0.27
>3 g/day	0.13	0.41

Source: Ripsin *et al.*, 1992.

that a substantial portion of the benefit is derived from the alcohol rather than other components of each type of drink (Rimm *et al.*, 1996).

6.4.10 Meal frequency

A series of experimental studies (Jenkins *et al.*, 1989; Arnold *et al.*, 1993; McGrath and Gibney, 1994) have each indicated that plasma total cholesterol and LDL-cholesterol can be reduced by an increase in meal frequency, the fall in cholesterol level of approximately 10% being of a similar order to that achieved by reduction in fat or saturates intake.

In the most recent study (McGrath and Gibney, 1994), in which individuals with a meal eating routine of about three meals a day increased to a snacking routine of about six meals a day and vice versa, plasma LDL-cholesterol fell by 0.4 mmol/l on moving from meal-eating to snacking and rose by 0.1 mmol/l when the switch was in the opposite direction.

These experimental studies are supported by a population based study of over 2000 men, aged 50–89 years, in which plasma total cholesterol was on average 0.2 mmol/l lower in those who ate four or more meals per day compared with those eating one or two meals daily. There was a difference of 0.16 mmol/l in LDL-cholesterol which persisted after adjustment for smoking, alcohol intake, waist-to-hip ratio, body mass index, systolic blood pressure and intake of all nutrients (Edelstein *et al.*, 1992).

Various mechanisms for the effect have been postulated. One suggestion is that frequent small meals cause more frequent and smaller rises in insulin and GIP (glucose-dependent insulinotropic polypeptide). The result of this could be an inhibition of the rate-limiting step in cholesterol synthesis via the regulating enzyme HMGCoA reductase. Small frequent fat intakes could also lead to frequent stimulation of reverse cholesterol transport, contributing to a reduction in plasma cholesterol by enhancing cholesterol breakdown (O'Flaherty and Gibney, 1994).

6.5 INFLUENCE OF DIETARY FACTORS ON PLASMA HOMOCYSTEINE

Folates, along with vitamin B6 and B12, play a key role in homocysteine metabolism. Homocysteine is either re-methylated to methionine in a reaction that requires methyl tetrahydrofolate and vitamin B12 as co-substrate and cofactor respectively, or metabolized to cysteine and α-ketobutyric acid in two successive vitamin B6 reactions.

Most individuals with increased levels of plasma homocysteine (Hcy) have suboptimal intakes of folate, vitamin B12 and vitamin B6 and supplementation with modest amounts of these vitamins results in a significant reduction in Hcy levels. Selhub *et al.* (1995) showed that suboptimal B vitamin status as well as increased levels of homocysteine were associated with increased likelihood of carotid artery stenosis.

In reviewing all the recent evidence relating Hcy to CHD, Stampfer and Malinow (1995) suggested that it was appropriate to make broad public health recommendations based on trials of secondary prevention and from disease progression data rather than wait for more expensive trials of primary prevention. In the meantime, they suggested that it would be prudent to ensure an adequate intake of folate. The mandatory folate fortification of cereal grain products in the USA which has been advocated to help reduce the number of births affected by neural tube defects was probably hastened by the evidence relating increased provision of folate to possible protection against CHD.

There is experimental evidence to suggest that by increasing dietary intake of folic acid (folate), and possibly other B vitamins such as B12, blood concentrations of homocysteine can be reduced. Theoretically, therefore, heart disease prevalence might be reduced by improved intakes of folate, found in foods such as leafy green vegetables, offal, bread, pulses and fortified breakfast cereals. In a recent paper, Boushey *et al.* (1995) attempted to assess the strength of the association between high homocysteine levels and coronary heart disease via a meta-analysis of relevant published studies, and to therefore assess the impact that dietary modification might have. Thirty-eight studies met their criteria, but only five of these included an association between CHD and dietary folate intakes as opposed to plasma folate levels, and no published studies have measured the effect of increasing dietary folate intake on risk of heart disease.

The meta-analysis revealed that for every 5 µmol/l increase in Hcy, men had a 1.6-fold increase in coronary heart disease risk and women a 1.8-fold increase. The associations also applied to stroke and peripheral vascular disease. In terms of its impact on cardiovascular risk, a 5 µmol/l increase in total blood Hcy is equivalent to an increase in blood cholesterol of 0.5 mmol/l. The authors estimated that increasing the daily intake of folic acid/folate by 200 µg should reduce homocysteine levels by about 4 µmol/l. On this basis, and assuming that reducing homocysteine level equates with reducing cardiovascular risk, 13 500–50 000 coronary deaths could be avoided annually. This fairly modest increase in folate could be achieved by dietary means – eating more green vegetables, pulses, cereal products and milk. It could also be achieved by expanding the range of foods fortified with folic acid. In fact, recent reports suggest that the folic acid that is present in fortified foods is better absorbed than naturally occurring folates (Cahill *et al.*, 1995; Cuskelly *et al.*, 1996). Before this benefit can be confirmed, however, a trial of folate/folic acid supplementation and its influence on homocysteine concentrations and coronary death rates is required.

6.6 INFLUENCE OF DIETARY FACTORS ON CLOTTING FACTORS INFLUENCING FIBRIN FORMATION AND DEPOSITION IN THE FIBROUS PLAQUE

Fibrin is formed from its precursor fibrinogen, and increased plasma fibrinogen concentration is an important risk factor for CHD. Fibrinogen concentration does not appear to be affected by dietary factors, with the possible exception of alcohol and perhaps, fish oils. The factors controlling the blood clotting mechanism are described in more detail in Chapters 2 and 3.

6.6.1 Alcohol

Although high alcohol intake is associated with increased BP and death from stroke, it is associated with decreased deaths from CHD (Figure 6.5). Moderate levels of alcohol intake (8–16 g or 1–2 units/day) appear to be protective against CHD. This is a real effect and not a statistical artefact due to the inclusion in the non-drinking category of people who have had to give up drinking due to ill-health (the so-called 'sick quitters').

The greater consumption of wine in France may be one explanation for the low rates of CHD compared with the UK, despite similar intakes of SFA in the two countries. Wine, however, may contain other protective factors, such as flavonoids, not found in other alcoholic drinks.

People who drink alcohol have lower plasma fibrinogen levels than non-drinkers, but it has not been demonstrated that increasing alcohol consumption leads to a reduction in fibrinogen levels. Higher intakes of alcohol are also associated with a reduced tendency for platelets to aggregate. Thus, alcohol might prevent thrombi deposition in the fibrous plaque by affecting both components of the blood clotting mechanism.

6.6.2 Fat

Total fat, rather than fatty acid composition, appears to have most influence on the clotting factor, Factor VII, which is a CHD risk factor. The effect appears to have two components: the first is the activation of the active enzyme by a high-fat meal; the second is the increase in the Factor VII precursor on a high-fat diet (Miller *et al.*, 1995).

There is also some evidence that a low intake of long-chain n-3 PUFA would raise fibrinogen levels and promote thrombi deposition in the fibrous plaque.

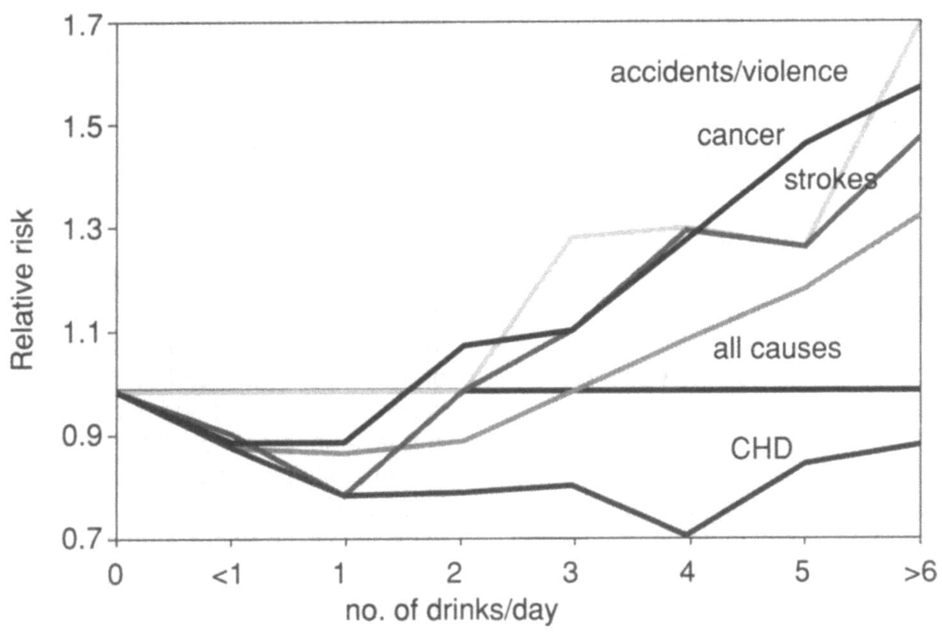

Figure 6.5 Alcohol consumption and relative risk of death over 12 years. (Source: Boffetta and Garfinkel, 1990.)

6.7 INSULIN RESISTANCE

6.7.1 Central fat distribution

(a) Evidence

Central fat distribution is strongly associated with a pattern of metabolic disorders termed the insulin resistance syndrome (Syndrome X). This involves the clustering of several CHD risk factors, including high BP, low plasma HDL-cholesterol, high fasting plasma triglyceride levels and increased plasma insulin. The mechanism is unknown but it may be related to the fact that the intra-abdominal fat depots release their fatty acids directly into the blood supply which goes to the liver.

Central fat distribution is associated with an increased risk of CHD. Men and women with pronounced central fat distribution have at least twice the risk of CHD as men and women with peripheral fat distribution (British Nutrition Foundation, 1992e).

Differences in fat distribution have been suggested as the main explanation for differences in CHD death rates between men and women. A man is about 3½ times more likely to get CHD than a pre-menopausal woman of the same age. Only a small proportion of this male–female difference in risk is due to the men having higher BP, higher plasma cholesterol levels or because they smoke more. On the other hand, a middle-aged woman with a 'central' distribution of body fat has roughly the same risk of developing CHD over the subsequent decade as a middle-aged man with a similar distribution.

Reducing central fat depots requires the same strategies as reducing weight in general, i.e. total energy input must be reduced below total energy output so that energy is drawn from fat stores. Studies using imaging techniques to give direct measures of internal fat depots have confirmed that, if anything, internal fats depots are mobilized in preference to external fat depots on weight loss and that they are not preferentially regained (van der Kooy, 1993; Ashwell, 1994).

(b) Proxy measures

Several proxy measures for central fat distribution have been suggested and the most popular in recent years has been the ratio of the waist circumference to the hip circumference (WHR). Recently, it has been suggested that the waist circumference alone (Han *et al.*, 1995; Lean *et al.*, 1995) or the ratio of waist circumference to height (WHTR) (Hseih and Yoshinaga, 1995; Ashwell *et al.*, 1996a; Cox *et al.*, 1996) are better proxy measures because they, like WHR, show associations with CHD risk factors which are usually stronger than those with Body Mass Index (BMI) (Manson *et al.*, 1995) but waist and WHTR are more suitable for use in a public health context.

(c) Possible mechanisms

Bjorntorp (1990) has suggested that central fat deposition can lead to an increase in risk factors for CHD because fatty acids are mobilized rapidly from the fat cells in certain central fat depots, primarily the omental and mesenteric depots, which are insensitive to insulin which usually acts to prevent fatty acid release. These fatty acids are released directly into the portal circulation where they stimulate increased VLDL production, increased glucose synthesis and decreased clearance of insulin. The net effect is an increase in triglyceride and LDL-cholesterol production.

Although there is no doubt that central obesity as measured by anthropometric indices is associated with increased deposition of internal fat depots, and although many studies have found direct associations between these depots as measured by computed tomography and by magnetic resonance imaging, there has been very little evidence to confirm or refute Bjorntorp's hypothesis. Again, WHTR is the anthropometric measure which shows strongest association with the total amount of intra-abdominal fat (Ashwell *et al.*, 1996b).

6.7.2 Non-starch polysaccharides

Ingestion of large quantities of certain soluble NSP can increase the viscosity of the luminal contents, thus reducing the speed at which the food travels along the intestine. This has the effect of reducing insulin resistance because the absorption of glucose – which acts as a stimulus to insulin release – takes place over a longer period.

6.7.3. Other influences

Insulin resistance can be reversed by weight loss and regular exercise. Altering dietary patterns (e.g. by spreading the total day's intake into several smaller meals) may also help.

6.8 INFLUENCE OF DIETARY FACTORS ON PLATELET AGGREGATION LEADING TO THROMBUS FORMATION (SEE FIGURE 6.6)

Measurement of the influence of diet on the tendency of blood to clot generally involves

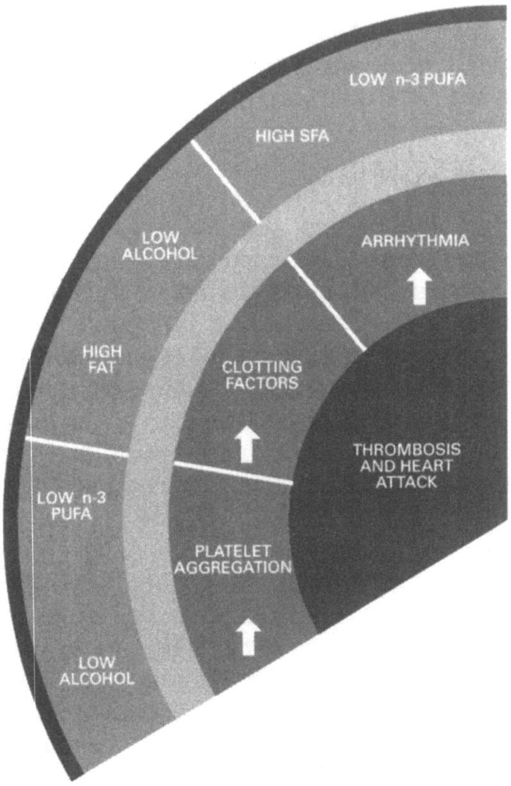

Figure 6.6 Dietary factors influencing physiological risk factors which lead to thrombosis and heart attack.

experimental measurement of constituent parts of the process:

- Platelets are stimulated to aggregate using various agents such as collagen. How readily this occurs can be measured in various ways.
- A small cut is made and the time for bleeding to stop is measured (the 'bleeding time').
- The amounts or activity of different factors in the coagulation 'cascade' are measured.
- The amounts or activity of the compounds controlling clot-dissolving (fibrinolysis) are measured.

None of these experimental measurements gives a completely accurate picture of the overall tendency for blood to coagulate in real life.

Dietary trials can be differentiated according to whether they involve the measurement of platelet responsiveness or bleeding time in people who are:

- naturally consuming different diets; or
- on experimental diets.

In the first case, other aspects of lifestyle, such as smoking, may provide confounding factors in large groups of people whereas in the second case, a much smaller group of people can be randomly allocated to diets. Although this provides the possibility for a double-blind, placebo-controlled trial, it does not accurately reflect real-life conditions.

6.8.1 n-3 Polyunsaturated fatty acids

Interest in the effects of n-3 PUFA began when Dyerberg and Bang (1979) compared Inuits (Eskimos) who have a relatively high n-3 PUFA consumption with Danes who have a low n-3 PUFA intake. Bleeding time was longer and the tendency for platelets to aggregate was reduced in the Inuits.

In Japan, platelet aggregation was reduced in the inhabitants of a fishing village who ate about 250 g fish per day, compared with farming villagers who ate about 90 g fish per day (Hirai *et al.*, 1982). In the Netherlands there were no differences in bleeding times or the tendency of platelets to aggregate between groups of people eating either 2 or 33 g of fish per day (Van Houwelingen *et al.*, 1989).

An intervention trial in the UK found that consumption of two portions of oil-rich fish each week by men who had already had one heart attack significantly reduced subsequent mortality from CHD over the next 2 years (Burr *et al.*, 1989). Deaths from CHD were reduced by 29% in the group given advice to eat fish compared with the group not

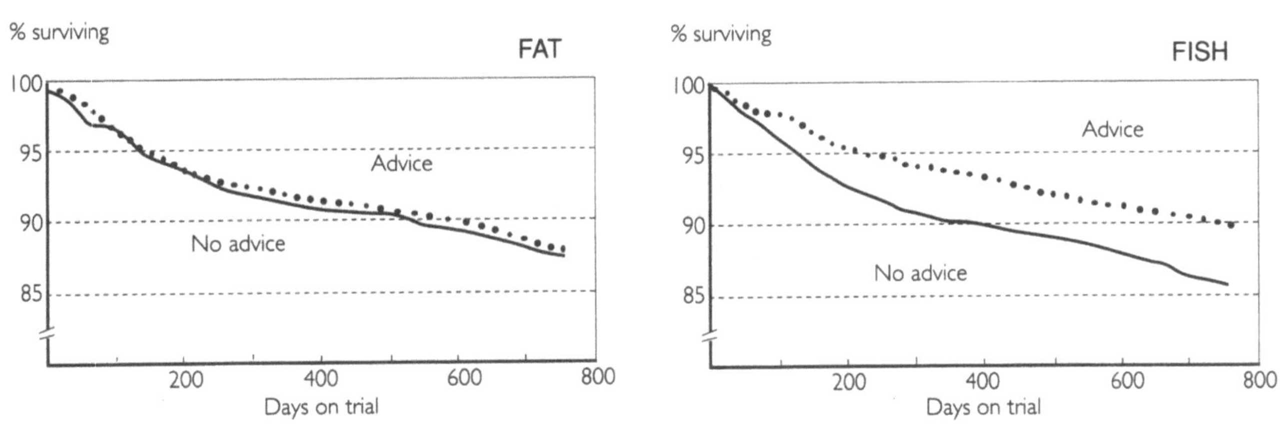

Figure 6.7 The beneficial effect of oil-rich fish on survival rates in the secondary prevention of CHD. (Source: Burr *et al.*, 1989.)

given advice (Figure 6.7). The total number of heart attacks in the two groups was not significantly different; however, fewer of them were fatal in the fish advice group.

In USA, the 6-year follow-up of the Health Professionals Study (Ascherio *et al.*, 1995) showed no association between intakes of n-3 fatty acids, adipose tissue levels of n-3 fatty acids, total fish intake and the incidence of CHD. However, the authors recognized the limitations of drawing conclusions from the study, namely:

- two-thirds of the men had greatly increased their intake of fish over the 10 years before 1986 (the baseline year for the study);
- fish intake in the educated health professionals was generally high; and
- the subjects were generally more health-conscious than average and the group with the high intakes of fish were taking other measures to reduce their CHD risk.

The overall conclusion is that eating oil-rich fish (about 200–300 g/day) results in prolonged bleeding times and reduced tendency for platelets to aggregate. The effect of eating 30 g/day or less (i.e. the amount that may be practical or acceptable in the UK) is uncertain. However, this more reasonable amount of fish consumption has been shown to be protective against a second heart attack.

The dietary factors responsible for the anti-coagulatory effects are thought to be n-3 PUFA such as EPA, which are present in marine oils. These replace the n-6 PUFA, arachidonic acid, in the platelet membrane, giving rise to thromboxanes which are much poorer stimulators of platelet aggregation than those derived from n-6 PUFA (see Figure 3.3).

However, it is possible to see diet-induced changes in the fatty acid composition of platelet membranes without parallel changes in platelet responsiveness. Furthermore, a reduced tendency for platelets to aggregate can persist for several weeks after stopping a diet high in fish oil.

6.8.2 Alcohol

There is some evidence that the platelets from people with increased frequency of alcohol consumption will have a reduced tendency to aggregate and that people who have had a heart attack are more likely to show increased platelet aggregation than those who have not (Renaud and de Lorgeril, 1992).

6.9 INFLUENCE OF DIETARY FACTORS ON CLOTTING FACTORS INFLUENCING FIBRIN FORMATION IN THE THROMBUS

There is preliminary evidence that moderate alcohol intake might inhibit the enzymes in the cascade leading to reduced fibrin formation and a reduced tendency for the blood to clot.

Most studies have found that fibrinogen concentration (see section 2.2.2) is unchanged by increasing dietary fish oils, although a small number have observed a reduction.

6.10 INFLUENCE OF DIETARY FACTORS ON ARRHYTHMIA

6.10.1 Saturated fatty acids

There is some evidence that diets with a high proportion of saturated fatty acids increase the tendency to cardiac arrhythmia. The SFA content of adipose tissue in men with serious arrhythmias who had recently had a heart attack was higher than in those not exhibiting arrhythmia.

6.10.2 n-3 Polyunsaturated fatty acids

Fish oil supplementation of the diet might reduce the severity of arrhythmias which occur during the period in which the heart muscle is starved of oxygen. This mechanism might explain why fish oil supplementation trials have shown no effect on non-fatal CHD events, while reducing CHD deaths.

The Lyon Diet Heart Study showed that a diet rich in α-linolenic acid as well as oleic acid and antioxidant nutrients was extremely effective in the secondary prevention of coronary events and death and raised the question of whether the high intake of α-linolenic acid (about 2 g/day) could have effects similar to those proposed for the long-chain n-3 PUFA. Compared with the DART trial, the Lyon protection extended to non-fatal MI and suggests that high intakes of α-linolenic acid might have an anti-arrhythmic effect as well as having effects via increased provision of the protective eicosanoids (de Lorgeril *et al.*, 1994).

In vitro studies of cultured heart cells suggest that the long-chain n-3 PUFA are modulating the calcium channels into the cells and thus helping to maintain a regular beat.

7

INTERACTIONS BETWEEN DIETARY COMPONENTS AND PHYSIOLOGICAL RISK FACTORS

Isolated examination of the effects on nutrients and their association with CHD risk is difficult, as factors tend to cluster together in dietary patterns, making the delineation of individual components, or even their cumulative effects, difficult to assess quantitatively.

One clear conclusion from a review of dietary factors is that the patterns of incidence of CHD cannot be attributed to any single factor. While each of the physiological conditions can individually increase the risk of CHD, the combination of different physiological conditions, dietary patterns and other lifestyle factors such as smoking have a greater effect than could be predicted from the sum of each individual effect acting alone.

Alternatively, the risk associated with a particular physiological condition, for example, increased LDL-cholesterol levels, may be reduced by the presence of a protective factor. These two types of interactions can be potentiating or protective.

7.1 POTENTIATING INTERACTIONS

A study of 126 middle-aged men in Finland found that the increase in thickness of the carotid artery wall over 2 years was accelerated in men with higher than average plasma LDL-cholesterol levels and higher than average plasma copper levels (Table 7.1). There was no accelerated increase in men with either high plasma LDL-cholesterol levels and low plasma copper levels, or high plasma copper levels and low plasma LDL-cholesterol levels (Salonen *et al.*, 1991).

The combination of high levels of LDL-cholesterol in a pro-oxidant environment is more likely to result in atherosclerotic thickening of the artery walls than high levels of LDL-cholesterol alone. The availability of copper in drinking water is enhanced by soft water. Copper pipes in soft water areas such as Glasgow may increase plasma copper concentrations.

Smoking, living in a soft water area with copper pipes, and a low fruit and vegetable intake may lead to a particularly deleterious combination of potentiating interactions.

High levels of plasma ferritin combined with high levels of LDL-cholesterol appear to put men at greater risk of CHD (Salonen *et al.*, 1992b). High levels of plasma ferritin in men with high levels of LDL-cholesterol were associated with an increased risk of heart attack of nearly five times the normal rate.

For men with low levels of LDL-cholesterol the increased risk associated with high levels of serum ferritin was less than two-fold. The combination of high levels of ferritin and LDL-cholesterol demonstrates another potentiating interaction.

There may be a potentiating interaction between low levels of vitamin E and plasma levels of other antioxidants. The Basel Study, monitoring disease in 3000 middle-aged men from whom blood samples had been obtained before any onset of disease symptoms, recorded an increased relative risk of subsequent CHD mortality in individuals with low plasma concentrations of vitamin C and carotene, regardless of vitamin E status.

These data have been used to suggest synergistic effects of both these nutrients against high plasma levels of vitamin E in relation to relative risk

Table 7.1 Increase in thickening of arterial wall (mm) after 2 years according to serum copper and LDL concentration

	Subjects with low LDL (<4.0 mmol/l)	**Subjects with high LDL** (≥4.0 mmol/l)
Low copper (<17.6 μmol/l)	0.08 mm	0.05 mm
High copper (≥17.6 μmol/l)	0.06 mm	0.25 mm

Source: Salonen *et al.*, 1991a.

Table 7.2 CHD deaths per 100 000 men in four selected communities according to plasma cholesterol and vitamin E status

Plasma cholesterol level	**Deaths**	
	Low-plasma vitamin E (<24 μmol/l)	**High plasma vitamin E** (>24 μmol/l)
(<6.0 mmol/l)	359 (SW Finland)	100 (Thun, Switzerland)
(>6.0 mmol/l)	381 (Glasgow)	186 (Schwedt, E Germany)

Source: Gey *et al.*, 1991.

of CHD. Thus, while data on lipid-standardized plasma vitamin E levels predicts 62 to 68% of the difference in CHD mortality between population groups, additional data on vitamin C and carotene increases the power of prediction to 88% (Gey *et al.*, 1991).

7.2 PROTECTIVE INTERACTIONS

Levels of plasma cholesterol in different European countries are relatively similar and yet rates of CHD vary seven-fold. In one study, high levels of plasma cholesterol were not associated with high rates of CHD if plasma levels of vitamin E were also high (Table 7.2).

A combination of high plasma cholesterol and low levels of plasma vitamin E (e.g. in Glasgow) resulted in higher rates of CHD than when both plasma cholesterol and vitamin E levels were high (Schwedt, East Germany).

A possible protective interaction between alcohol and fat has been proposed to explain the low rate of CHD in France and the higher than expected rates in the UK despite similar levels of plasma cholesterol and intakes of dairy fats in the two countries. If wine consumption is also taken into account, the rates of CHD in France and the UK are closer to those predicted from observed risk factors (Renaud and de Lorgeril, 1992).

Protective interactions should also be considered in dietary manipulation to reduce risk factors.

The addition of fish oil to diets has been shown to enhance the effects of dietary sodium restriction in reducing BP in elderly people (Cobiac *et al.*, 1991). Many studies examining the addition of fish oil into diets indicate modest reductions in BP in subjects with raised BP, but larger reductions cannot be achieved. The interactive effects of fish oil and sodium restriction are likely to produce greater reductions in BP than either factor alone.

A stronger combined effect on blood lipids has also been observed when soluble NSP (Chapter 6) was added to diets. Jenkins *et al.* (1993) observed additional reductions in total cholesterol levels and levels of LDL and HDL-cholesterol in subjects on base-line diets with low intakes (less than 4% of energy) from SFA after addition of high levels of soluble NSP, mainly as legumes, oat bran and psyllium-enriched breakfast cereals.

Again, recommendations for dietary manipulation could consider the greater potency of influencing risk factors where there may be synergistic interactions between dietary factors.

8

WHAT DIETARY CHANGES ARE NECESSARY TO REDUCE CORONARY HEART DISEASE?

8.1 CHANGES TO THE NUTRIENT COMPOSITION OF THE DIET

8.1.1 Fats

The Government White Paper 'The Health of the Nation' (Department of Health, 1992) set targets for the reduction of deaths from CHD in England and Wales and the strategies by which it is hoped to achieve them. The targets proposed are the reduction of premature deaths (under 65 years) by at least 40% and the reduction of deaths in the age-range 65–74 years by at least 30% in the year 2000 from baseline figures in 1990.

The dietary strategies proposed to support these targets are the reduction in the percentage of energy from total fat and SFA to the levels proposed in the Dietary Reference Value (DRV) Report (Department of Health, 1991), i.e. 33% and 10% of total dietary energy, respectively. (The level for total fat is derived from the summation of DRVs for individual classes of fatty acids plus glycerol.)

Population average intakes of SFA in 1986/7 were 15.4% of total energy in men and 16.5% in women (Gregory *et al.*, 1990). Present levels of plasma cholesterol are on average 5.8 mmol/l. It has been calculated that reducing SFA intakes to 10% of total dietary energy should lower average plasma cholesterol levels by 0.4 mmol/l, resulting in average levels of 5.4 mmol/l.

Plasma cholesterol levels would be most effectively lowered by reducing intakes of SFA that have most effect on cholesterol levels. Myristic acid (14 : 0) and lauric acid (12 : 0) are the most potent but they are only found in significant quantities in dairy fats and coconut oil. Palmitic acid (16 : 0) is less potent but is much more widespread in foods.

The DRV Report proposed that PUFA should continue to provide a population average intake of 6% of total dietary energy from a mixture of n-6 and n-3 PUFA, that *cis*-MUFA should continue to provide 12% of dietary energy and *trans* fatty acids no more than 2% of dietary energy. The report cautioned against an increase in consumption of any fatty acid, and advised that intakes of PUFA should not exceed 10% of dietary energy in any individual as a caution against increased oxidation of tissue lipids. In the light of further evidence, the BNF Task Force on Unsaturated Fatty Acids (British Nutrition Foundation, 1992d) recommended that population average intakes of the long-chain n-3 PUFA should increase substantially to 0.5% of total energy.

The report of the Cardiovascular Review Group (the 1994 CRG Report) on *Nutritional Aspects of Cardiovascular Disease* (Department of Health, 1994) reiterated the recommendations in the DRV report for average intakes of total fat, saturated fatty acids and polyunsaturated fatty acids. It made no specific recommendations for monounsaturates but did comment that they might usefully substitute for saturates within an overall fat ceiling.

The Report also recommended an increase in the population average consumption of long-chain n-3 PUFA, but one which was more conservative than the BNF recommendation – from about 0.1 g/day to 0.2 g/day (1.5 g/week).

The 1994 CRG Report made the first UK recommendation about dietary cholesterol and said that the average intake, which is about 245 mg/day, should not rise.

The Report also reiterated the recommendation in the DRV Report that, on average, *trans* fatty acids should provide no more than the current average of about 2% of dietary energy and specified 'that consideration should be given to ways of decreasing the amount present in the diet'.

The British Nutrition Foundation's Task Force on *trans* Fatty Acids (British Nutrition Foundation, 1995a) also concluded that it would be prudent not to let average intakes of *trans* fatty acids rise.

8.1.2 Starches and non-starch polysaccharides

The DRV Report recommended increases in population average intakes of starch and NSP. Population average NSP intakes should increase to 18 g/day (with an individual maximum intake of 24 g) and starches along with intrinsic and milk sugars should provide approximately 37% of dietary energy intakes.

This should be achieved by increasing starch

intakes to about one-third of energy requirements. Obtaining more energy from starch is also a means of decreasing consumption of other nutrients, particularly fat and sugars.

The 1994 CRG Report introduced the term 'complex carbohydrates' to cover starch and NSP and recommended that complex carbohydrates, and sugars in fruit and vegetables, should restore the energy deficit following a reduction in the dietary intake of fat. The Report recommended that the proportion of dietary energy derived from carbohydrates should increase to approximately 50%. It reiterated the DRV Report's recommendation for an increase in NSP intakes and said that the average intake from non-milk extrinsic sugars should not contribute more than about 10% of energy, mainly because of undesirable effects on dental health, rather than any effect on CHD.

8.1.3 Sodium and potassium

Intakes of salt (from foods and discretionary additions of salt in cooking and at the table) were estimated in 1986/7 to be about 10.3 g/day in men and 7.2 g/day in women (3.37 and 2.35 g of sodium respectively).

The 1991 DRV Report considered current intakes of sodium in the UK to be needlessly high and cautioned against any increase, while accepting that possible public health benefits such as reduced cardiovascular mortality may accompany reductions in population sodium intakes. Although DRVs were set for sodium and potassium on the basis of physiological needs, there were no recommendations for average intakes. The 1994 CRG Report, however, did make specific recommendations for reducing average intakes of sodium and increasing average intakes of potassium (see section 8.2.3).

8.1.4 Antioxidants

Traditionally, reference values for micronutrients have been developed to ensure that the nutritional needs of practically all healthy persons in a population are met. Specific benefits of values above reference intakes for sub-groups of the population have often been referred to in discussion within background literature for official figures. However, acceptance of higher intakes for some sections of the population have not been given formal status other than for pregnant and lactating women.

The most recent review of micronutrient requirements for the UK population was documented in the DRV Report (Department of Health, 1991). The views of the DRV Panel in relation to antioxidant vitamins were set out within relevant sections for each nutrient:

(a) Carotenoids

The proposed role for these pigments as active antioxidants in tissues deactivating free radicals was acknowledged, although the DRV Panel considered the evidence insufficient to make recommendations for intakes beyond their role as precursors for vitamin A.

About 75% of current intakes of retinol equivalents in the UK diet is supplied by pre-formed retinol, the remaining 25% of vitamin A activity coming from carotenoids (mainly β-carotene) (see Chapter 5). Future assessments of nutrient requirements may need to differentiate the pro-vitamin A activities of the carotenoids from specific activities contributing to antioxidant potential, and thus to define separate reference intakes for carotenoids or dietary carotenoid/retinol ratios.

The US review of Recommended Dietary Allowances issued in 1989 (National Research Council, 1989) also referred to current evidence supporting the specific roles of carotenoids other than their pro-vitamin A activity. While no specific level or intake was proposed, the report concluded that the evidence suggests some benefit from generous intakes of carotenoid-rich foods.

(b) Vitamin C

The antioxidant capabilities of ascorbic acid were referred to, but not considered in detail by the DRV Panel. Reference intakes were formulated on the basis of ensuring a body pool size sufficient to provide at least 1 month's safety interval on zero intake before any evidence of impaired function.

From these data, average requirements for men and women (15 years plus) were considered to be 25 mg/day, the higher reference nutrient intake of 40 mg/day being considered adequate to ensure that requirements for 97.5% of the healthy population are met. Specific reference to higher requirements in smokers was made along with possible risks associated with high intakes of vitamin C.

(c) Vitamin E

The DRV Panel felt that there were insufficient data in the literature to indicate specific reference levels for this vitamin, although a figure for a 'safe intake' was proposed at above 3 mg/day for women and 4 mg/day for men. A further provision for infants at 0.4 mg vitamin E per gram PUFA was also defined.

In view of considerable current data indicating an association between diets generally higher in the antioxidant nutrients, and the lower incidence of certain chronic diseases including CHD, future policy documents may consider the provision of additional data on antioxidant micronutrient intakes to include parameters for intakes which cover more than physiological requirements that may benefit population sub-groups. However, the inconsistent evidence emerging from the antioxidant intervention trials (see section 6.2.3) will make this task more difficult than it appeared a few years ago.

(d) Antioxidants in foods or as dietary supplements?

The 1994 CRG Report (Department of Health, 1994) considered that its recommendation for an increase in starchy foods and fruits and vegetables and substitution of unsaturated vegetable oils for more saturated animal fats would have the effect of increasing the consumption of various antioxidants, including vitamin C, vitamin E, carotenoids and polyphenolic compounds such as flavonoids. It did not recommend supplementation with concentrated or purified preparations as a widespread policy for CHD prevention, as long-term safety and efficacy in a variety of populations had not been demonstrated. In contrast, a diet rich in vegetables and fruits is generally regarded as conducive to long-term health.

8.2 THE FOODS WE EAT

8.2.1 Fats

A reduction in fat from full-fat dairy products is likely to lead to a greater fall in plasma cholesterol levels than an equivalent reduction in total fat from meat products such as pies, sausages and burgers.

The 1994 CRG Report (Department of Health, 1994) has recommended that 'people use reduced fat spreads and dairy products instead of full fat products'. It also recommended that 'people replace fats rich in saturated fatty acids with oils and fats low in saturated fatty acids and rich in monounsaturated fatty acids'.

In order to achieve a substantial increase in n-3 PUFA, the British Nutrition Foundation Task Force on Unsaturated Fatty Acids (1992d) recommended eating between one and three portions a week of oil-rich fish such as pilchards, herring, mackerel and salmon.

The 1994 CRG Report made a slightly more conservative recommendation that 'people should eat at least two portions of fish, of which one should be oily fish, weekly'.

8.2.2 Starches and non-starch polysaccharides

The reduction in fat will require an increase in the intakes of carbohydrates in order to compensate for the reduction in energy intakes in non-obese subjects. The recommended increase in population average intakes of NSP supports the particular place of starchy foods in the achievement of dietary targets. Increased consumption of fruits and vegetables and of starchy staple foods (bread, rice, potatoes, pasta) are likely to have multiple dietary benefits.

The 1994 CRG Report recommended that 'the consumption of vegetables, fruit, potatoes and bread should be increased by at least 50%'.

8.2.3 Sodium and potassium

A reduction in sodium (salt) intakes is best achieved by a reduction in the use of discretionary salt added to foods during domestic preparation or at the table, and also a reduction in sodium-containing foods. Bread is currently an important dietary contributor to average sodium intake but because of its benefit as a starchy food, a reduction in other salt-containing foods would be preferable to achieve the desired effect on average salt intakes.

A gradual reduction in the sodium content of processed foods is a further approach. As it would take some time for people to become accustomed to low-salt bread and breakfast cereals, a small-step over time may be the most effective strategy. A concerted communication effort would be needed to encourage people to be more receptive to small taste changes in standard products.

The use of 'salt-substitutes' (non- or low-sodium salts) may have a particularly useful role in enhancing the palatability of low-sodium therapeutic diets prescribed in cases with diagnosed hypertension.

Fresh fruits and vegetables have a low sodium/potassium ratio, and increasing consumption of these would increase potassium intake, improving the sodium/potassium ratio of the diet.

The 1994 CRG Report recommended 'a reduction in the average intake of sodium (principally from common salt (sodium chloride)) by the adult population from the current level of about 150 mmol/day (equivalent to 9 g salt/day) to about 100 mmol/day (6 g salt/day) and an increase in the average intake of potassium by the adult population to about 3.5 g/day (90 mmol/day)'. It also recommended a similar proportionate reduction in the sodium content and a similar proportionate increase in the potassium content of children's diets, but said 'there was insufficient data to quantify this'.

The Report also recommended that food manufacturers, caterers and individuals should 'explore and grasp the opportunities for reducing the sodium content of foods and meals'.

The recommendation for an average reduction of about one-third in salt intakes was not universally accepted by some sectors of the food industry and similar sentiments were expressed as those to a similar recommendation from WHO (1994): 'The wisdom of this advice is still debated but the evidence is good enough to suggest that some (salt) reduction ***together with*** other proposed dietary changes and weight reduction in the overweight, could reduce BP and ultimately help to achieve *The Health of the Nation* CHD targets' (British Nutrition Foundation, 1994).

8.2.4 Fruit and vegetables

Initial studies indicate a consistent protective association between CHD and the consumption of fruits and vegetables in amounts higher than would be required to ensure the provision of intakes of vitamins set out in the various reports on nutrient requirements (National Research Council, 1989; Department of Health, 1991).

It is probable that antioxidant activity is attributable to both nutrient and non-nutrient components commonly found in fruits and vegetables. A considerable increase in the consumption of this group of foods is likely to improve many nutritional parameters, including the intake of antioxidants.

Low intakes of fruits and vegetables are more commonly seen in men, particularly in the North and Scotland, and generally in children and younger adults. The average intake of fruits and vegetables in 1986/7 was 200–250 g/day (Gregory *et al.*, 1990).

In 1990, the World Health Organization recommended a population nutrient goal of 400 g of fruit and vegetables (excluding tubers), including at least 30 g of pulses, nuts and seeds. No upper limit was set. The 400 g goal was 'judgementally', based on apparently healthy fruit and vegetables intakes in countries with low rates of CHD.

The 1994 CRG Report made a recommendation that fruit and vegetable consumption should increase by 50%, based on the Panel's assessment of a feasible dietary change for the UK, and not necessarily on what may lead to the lowest attainable rate for CHD. To achieve this increase would require a total intake of approximately six portions of vegetables or fruit. This recommendation was subsequently reiterated in *The Balance of Good Health* (HEA, 1994) but this time it was rephrased to recommend intakes of five or more portions a day of fruit and vegetables. Williams (1995) has summarized some practical suggestions of how this advice can be put into practice.

The 1994 CRG Report advice to increase current intakes of fruit and vegetables by 50% would raise levels of vitamin C and carotene to levels similar to those of the top one-fifth of the UK population. This could raise vitamin C intakes to around 110 mg and β-carotene intakes to about 4 mg/day, but it would not have much effect on vitamin E levels.

Advice on eating more fruit and vegetables might have to be more specific and emphasize choosing fruits and vegetables which are particularly good sources of carotenoids and flavonoids such as carrots, peppers, onions and green leafy vegetables such as broccoli. The simple 'fruits and vegetables' message would still not help to achieve an increase in vitamin E and this would have to come from eating more wholegrain cereal and margarines and oils rich in polyunsaturated fatty acids.

8.2.5 Alcohol

After reviewing the scientific evidence relating alcohol consumption to CHD, The Inter-Departmental Working Group On Sensible Drinking (DH, 1995a) made the following recommendations:

- 'The health benefit from drinking relates to men aged over 40 (and post-menopausal women) and the major part of this can be obtained at levels as low as 1 unit a day with the maximum health advantage lying between 1 and 2 units a day'.
- 'Regular consumption of between 3 and 4 units a day by men (2 and 3 units a day by women) of all ages will not accrue significant health risk'.
- 'Consistently drinking 4 or more units a day by men (3 or more units a day by women) is not advised as a sensible drinking level because of the progressive health risk it carries'.

8.3 THE WHOLE DIET

Eight Guidelines for a Healthy Diet (MAFF, DH, HEA, 1990) summarized the main nutrition education messages of the Dietary Reference Values report for professionals, and materials such as *Enjoy Healthy Eating* (HEA, 1991) provided practical advice for use with and by the public about choosing a healthy diet, based on these messages. The Guidelines are:

1. Enjoy your food
2. Eat a variety of different foods
3. Eat the right amount to be a healthy weight
4. Eat plenty of foods rich in starch and fibre

5. Don't eat too much fat
6. Don't eat sugary foods too often
7. Look after the vitamins and minerals in your food
8. If you drink alcohol, keep within sensible limits

The *Balance of Good Health* (HEA, 1994) was the name given to the National Food Guide which was based on the Government's Eight Guidelines for a Healthy Diet. It aims to make healthy eating easier to understand by showing the types and proportions of foods needed to make a well-balanced and healthy diet. It divides food into five food groups and gives the following advice on how much to choose:

1. Bread, other cereals and potatoes – eat lots
2. Fruit and vegetables – eat lots
3. Milk and dairy foods – eat or drink moderate amounts and choose lower fat versions whenever you can
4. Meat, fish and alternatives – eat moderate amounts and choose lower fat versions whenever you can
5. Foods containing fat and foods containing sugar – eat foods containing fat sparingly and choose lower fat versions. Foods containing sugar should not be eaten too often as they can contribute to tooth decay.

The 1994 CRG Report noted that 'the nutrient content of the average diet in Britain differs in a number of respects from that recommended in the Report' and said 'there are as many different ways of responding to the recommendations as there are individual diets'. It seems likely that any changes in the national pattern of consumption would result from a variety of changes across the whole range of foodstuffs rather than drastic changes in one or two. 'On this assumption the population as a whole would consume less fatty meat and meat products, high-fat dairy products and full-fat spreads, etc. In addition, lower-fat and lower-salt versions of more foods would need to be developed and little salt added to food "at table". A substantial increase would take place in the average amount of potatoes, bread, pasta and other carbohydrate-rich foods eaten, in order to replace the energy that would be lost if fat intake was reduced.'

With the profusion of advice about the composition of a 'healthy balanced diet', it is particularly important that the first two of the *Eight Guidelines for a Healthy Diet* do not get overlooked. 'Enjoy your food and eat a variety of different foods' is still probably the best and simplest advice that can be given on the subject of diet and the way it can protect against heart disease.

9

CONCLUSIONS

Dietary advice for the general population should include encouragement to eat a great variety of fruit and vegetables, more starchy foods such as potatoes, rice, bread and pasta, and more oil-rich fish. Regular, light drinking should also be encouraged in men aged over 40 years and in post-menopausal women. Advice should also be given to eat more reduced fat rather than full-fat dairy products and full-fat meat products, and to use less salt. Special emphasis should be put on the importance of enjoying all food and eating a wide variety of different foods.

The proposed reduction in plasma cholesterol levels from such dietary changes, if achieved, has been estimated to result in, at most, a 15–20% reduction in CHD deaths. The Round Table Model has emphasized that plasma cholesterol is just one of the factors leading to an adverse lipid profile which, in turn, is one of the many physiological risk factors leading to CHD. However, this dietary advice is appropriate for the reduction of other risk factors, such as reducing blood pressure and reducing platelet aggregation.

Dietary advice to the general population, though, should always be part of a package which includes advice to stop smoking, to take more exercise, to maintain a healthy weight, and also to relieve stress.

REFERENCES

Addis, P.B. and Park, S.W. (1988) Role of lipid oxidation products in atherosclerosis. In *Food Toxicology* (eds S.L. Tayler and R.A. Scanlen), IFT, Basic Symposium Series, Dekker, New York.

Albanes, D. and Heinonen, O. (The Alpha-Tocopherol, Beta Carotene Cancer Prevention Study Group) (1994) The effect of vitamin E and beta carotene on the incidence of lung cancer and other cancers in male smokers. *N. Engl. J. Med.* **330**, 15: 1029–1035.

Anderson, K.M., Wilson, W.F., Odell, P.M. *et al.* (1991) An updated coronary risk profile. AHA statement. *Circulation*, **83**: 356–362.

Arnold, L.M. *et al.* (1993) Effect of isoenergetic intake of three or nine meals on plasma lipoproteins and glucose metabolism. *Am. J. Clin. Nutr.*, **57**: 446–451.

Ascherio, A., Rimm, E.B., Stampfer, M.J. *et al.* (1995) Dietary intake of marine n-3 fatty acids, fish intake, and the risk of coronary disease among men. *N. Engl. J. Med.*, **332**: 977–982.

Ashwell, M. (1996) Leaping into shape. In *Bodyweight and Health* (ed M.J. Sadler). Proceedings of the British Nutrition Foundation conference, British Nutrition Foundation, London: 47–54.

Ashwell, M. and Buss, D. (1995) Vitamin intake in Great Britain: Association with Mortality rates for coronary heart disease. In *The Scientific Basis for Vitamin Intake in Human Nutrition* (ed. P. Walter), Bibl Nutr Dieta, Karger, Basel: 128–136.

Ashwell, M.A., Lejeune, S.R.E. and McPherson, K. (1996a) Ratio of waist circumference to height may be a better indicator of need for weight management. *Br. Med. J.*, **312**: 377.

Ashwell, M.A, Cole, T.J. and Dixon, A.K. (1996b) Ratio of waist circumference : height is a strong predictor of intra-abdominal fat. *Br. Med. J.* (in press).

Barker, D.J.P. (1991) Programming of cardiovascular disease in fetal life and infancy. *BNF Nutr. Bull.*, **16 (Suppl)**: 29–37.

Barker, D.J.P. (1994) *Mothers, Babies and Disease in Later Life*, BMJ Publishing Group, London.

Barker, D.J.P. (1995a) Fetal origins of coronary heart disease. *Br. Med. J.*, **311**: 171–174.

Barker, D.J.P. (1995b) The fetal and infant origins of disease. *Eur. J.Clin. Invest.*, **25**: 457–463.

Bartley, M. *et al.* (1994) Birthweight and later socio-economic disadvantage: evidence from the 1958 British cohort study. *Br. Med. J.*, **309**: 1475–1479.

Bennett, N., Dodd, T., Flatley, J., Freeth, S. and Bolling, K. (1995) *Health Survey for England, 1993*, HMSO, London.

Berg, K. (1985) Genetics of coronary heart disease. In *Progress in Medical Genetics, Vol. V* (eds A.G. Steinberg, A.G. Bearn, A.G. Motulsky and B. Childs), WB Saunders Co., Philadelphia: 35–90.

Berg, K. (1991) Interaction of nutrition and genetic factors in health and disease. Proceedings of 6th European Nutrition Conference. *Eur. J. Clin. Nutr.*, **45 (Suppl. 2)**: 8–13.

Berry, E.M., Hirsch, J., Most, J., McNamara, D.J. and Thornton, J. (1986) The relationship of dietary fat to plasma lipid levels as studied by factor analysis of adipose tissue composition in a free-living population of middle-aged American men. *Am. J. Clin. Nutr.*, **44**: 220–231.

Bjorntorp, P. (1990) Portal adipose tissue as a generator of risk factors for cardiovascular disease and diabetes. *Arteriosclerosis*, **10**: 493–496.

Boffetta, P. and Garfinkel, L. (1990) Alcohol drinking and mortality among men enrolled in an American Cancer Society prospective study. *Epidemiology*, **1**: 342–348.

Boushey, C.J., Beresford, S.A.A., Omenn, G.S. *et al.* (1995) A quantitative assessment of plasma homocysteine as a risk factor for vascular disease. *JAMA*, **274**: 1049–1057.

British Nutrition Foundation (1987) *Task Force Report. Trans fatty acids*, BNF, London.

British Nutrition Foundation (1990) *Task Force Report. Complex carbohydrates*, Chapman & Hall, London.

British Nutrition Foundation (1991) *Antioxidant nutrients in health and disease*. Briefing paper no. 25, BNF, London.

British Nutrition Foundation (1992a) *Coronary heart disease – I: The wider perspective.* Briefing paper no. 26, BNF, London.

British Nutrition Foundation (1992b) *Coronary heart disease – 2: What is it and what are the uncontrollable factors?* Briefing paper no. 28, BNF, London.

British Nutrition Foundation (1992c) *Coronary heart disease – 3: The role of dietary fats.* Briefing paper no. 29, BNF, London.

British Nutrition Foundation (1992d) *Task Force Report. Unsaturated Fatty Acids: Nutritional and Physiological Significance*, Chapman & Hall, London.

British Nutrition Foundation (1992e) *The nature and risks of obesity.* Briefing paper no. 27, BNF, London.

British Nutrition Foundation (1993) *Diet and Heart Disease*, BNF, London.

British Nutrition Foundation (1994) *Salt in the diet.* Briefing paper, BNF, London.

British Nutrition Foundation (1995a) *Task Force Report. Trans Fatty Acids.* British Nutrition Foundation, London.

British Nutrition Foundation (1995b) *Task Force Report. Iron. Nutritional and Physiological Significance.* Chapman & Hall, London.

Brown, A. (1992) Oxidatively-modified lipoproteins in coronary heart disease. *BNF Nutr. Bull.*, **17 (Suppl.)**: 49–64.

Brunner, E. (1995) *Is stress a factor in coronary heart disease?* Family Heart Association, Oxford.

Burr, M.L., Fehily, A.M., Gilbert, J.F. *et al.* (1989) Effects of changes in fat, fish and fibre intakes on death and myocardial reinfarction; diet and reinfarction trial (DART). *Lancet*, **2**: 757–761.

Cahill, E. (1995) Iron and folic acid nutrition in women of reproductive age. PhD thesis, University of Dublin Trinity College.

Cambien, F., Jacqueson, A., Richard, J.L., Warnet, J.M., Ducimetiere, P. and Claude, J.K. (1986) Is the level of serum triglyceride a sufficient predictor of coronary death in 'normal cholesterolaemic' subjects? The Paris Prospective Study. *Am. J. Epidemiol.*, **124**: 624–632.

Castelli, W.P., Doyle, J.T. and Gordon, T. (1977) Alcohol and blood lipids. The cooperative lipoprotein physiotyping study. *Lancet*, **ii**: 153–155.

Chamberlain, J.C. and Galton, D.J. (1990) Genetic susceptibility to atherosclerosis. In *Lipids and Cardiovascular Disease* (eds D.J. Galton and G.R. Thompson), Churchill Livingstone, Edinburgh.

Cobiac, L., Martel, P., Wing, L. and Howe, P. (1991) The effects of dietary sodium restriction and fish oil supplementation on blood pressure in the elderly. *Clin. Exp. Pharmacol. Physiol.*, **18**: 265–268.

Collins, R., Peto, R., MacMahon, S. *et al.* (1990) Blood pressure, stroke and coronary heart disease. Part 2, Short term reductions in blood pressure: overview of randomised drug trials in their epidemiological context. *Lancet*, 335: 827–838.

Cox, B.D., Whichelow, M.J., Ashwell, M. and Prevost, A.T. (1996) Comparison of anthropometric indices as predictors of mortality in British adults. *Int. J.Obesity*, **20 (Suppl. 4)**: 141.

Cox, C., Mann, J., Sutherland, W. *et al.* (1995) Individual variation in plasma cholesterol response to dietary saturated fat. *Br. Med. J.*, **311**: 1260–1264.

Cuskelly, G.J., McNulty, H. and Scott, J.M. (1996) Effect of increasing dietary folate on red-cell folate: implications for prevention of neural tube defects. *Lancet*, **347**: 657–659.

Davey Smith, G. and Pekkanen, J. (1992) Should there be a moratorium on the use of cholesterol-lowering drugs? *Br. Med. J.*, **304**: 431–434.

Davey Smith, G., Song, F. and Sheldon, T.A. (1993) Cholesterol lowering and mortality: the importance of considering initial level of risk. *Br. Med. J.*, **306**: 1367–1373.

Dayton, S., Pearce, M.L., Hashimoto, S., Dixon, W.J. and Tomiyasu, U. (1969) A controlled clinical trial of a diet high in unsaturated fat in preventing complications of atherosclerotic complications. *Circulation*, **60 (Suppl. 2)**: 1–63.

de Lorgeril, M., Renaud, S., Mamelle, N. *et al.* (1994) Mediterranean alpha-linolenic acid-rich diet in secondary prevention of coronary heart disease. *Lancet*, **343**: 1454–1459.

Den Heijer, M., Blom, H.J., Gerrits, W.B.J. *et al.* (1995) Is hyperhomocysteinaemia a risk factor for recurrent venous thrombosis? *Lancet*, **345**: 882–885.

Department of Health (1991) Report on Health and Social Subjects No. 41. Dietary reference values for food energy and nutrients for the United Kingdom. Committee on Medical Aspects of Food Policy. HMSO, London.

Department of Health (1992) *The Health of the Nation.* HMSO, London.

Department of Health (1994) *Nutritional Aspects of Cardiovascular Disease.* Report on Health and Social Subjects No. 46, HMSO, London.

Department of Health (1995a) *Sensible drinking.* The Report of an Inter-Departmental Working group. Department of Health, London.

Department of Health (1995b) *Obesity. Reversing the Increasing problem of obesity in England.* A report from the Nutrition and Physical Activity Task Forces.

Dyerberg, J. and Bang, H.O. (1979) Haemostatic function and platelet polyunsaturated fatty acids in Eskimos. *Lancet*, **2**: 433–435.

Edelstein, S.L. *et al.* (1992) Increased meal frequency associated with decreased cholesterol concentration. *Am. J. Clin. Nutr.*, **55**: 664–669.

Fehily, A.M., Yarnell, J.W.G., Bolton, C.H. and Butland, B.K. (1988) Dietary determinants of plasma lipids and lipoproteins; the Caerphilly Study. *Eur. J. Clin. Nutr.*, **42**: 405–413.

Felton, C.V., Crook, D., Davies, M.J. *et al.* (1994) Dietary polyunsaturated fatty acids and composition of human aortic plaques. *Lancet*, **344**: 1195–1196.

Fleck, A. (1989) Latitude and ischaemic heart disease. *Lancet*, **1**: 613.

Frankel, E.N., Kanner, J., German, J.B., Parko, E. and Kinsella, J.E. (1993) Inhibition of oxidation of human low-density lipoprotein by phenolic substances in red wine. *Lancet*, **341**: 454–457.

Frantz, I.D., Dawson, E.A., Ashman, P.L. *et al.* (1989) Test of effect of lipid lowering by diet on cardiovascular risk. *Arteriosclerosis*, **9**: 129–135.

Frick, M.H., Elo, O., Haapa, K. *et al.* (1987) Helsinki heart study: primary prevention trial with gemfibrozil in middle-aged men with dyslipidaemia. *N. Engl. J. Med.*, **317**: 1237–1245.

Fuchs, C.S., Stampher, M.J., Colditz, G.A. *et al.* (1995) Alcohol consumption and mortality among women. *N. Engl. J. Med.*, **332**: 1245–1250.

Fuster, V., Budimon, L., Budimon, J.J. and Chesebro, J.H. (1992) The pathogenesis of coronary artery disease and the acute coronary syndromes. *N. Engl. J. Med.*, **326**: 242–249, 310–318.

Gey, F.K., Puska, P., Jordan, P. and Moser, U.K. (1991) Inverse correlation between plasma vitamin E and mortality from ischaemic heart disease in cross-cultural epidemiology. *Am. J. Clin. Nutr.*, **53**: 326S–334S.

Gintner, E. (1995) Cardiovascular risk factors in the former communist countries. Analysis of 40 European MONICA populations. *Eur. J. Epidemiol.*, **11**: 199–205.

Gordon, D.J., Probstfield, T.H., Garnson, R.J. *et al.* (1989) HDL cholesterol and cardiovascular disease. Four prospective American studies. *Circulation*, **74**: 8–15.

Gregory, J., Foster, K., Tyler, H. and Wiseman, M. (1990) *The dietary and nutritional survey of British adults*. HMSO, London.

Grundy, S.M. (1988) Cholesterol and heart disease: a new era. *J. Am. Med. Assoc.*, **256**: 2849–2858.

Grundy, S.M. and Denke, M.A. (1990) Dietary influences on serum lipids and lipoproteins. *J. Lipid Res.*, **31**: 1149–1172.

Han, T.S., van Leer, E.M., Seidell, J.C. and Lean, M.E.J. (1995) Waist circumference action levels in the identification of cardiovascular risk factors: prevalence study in a random sample. *Br. Med. J.*, **311**: 1401–1405.

Hayes, K.C. and Khosla, P. (1992) Dietary fatty acid thresholds and cholesterolaemia. *FASEB J.*, **6**: 2600–2607.

HEA (1991) *Enjoy Healthy Eating*, HEA, London.

HEA (1994) *The Balance of Good Health*, HEA, London.

Hegsted, D.M., Aksman, L., Johnson, J.A. *et al.* (1993) Dietary fat and serum lipids: an evaluation of the experimental data. *Am. J. Clin. Nutr.*, **57**: 875–883.

Hein, H.O., Suadicani, P. and Gyntelberg, F. (1996) Alcohol consumption, serum low density lipoprotein cholesterol concentration, and risk of ischaemic heart disease: six year follow up in the Copenhagen male study. *Br. Med. J.*, **312**: 736–741.

Hennekens, C.H., Buring, J.E., Manson, J.E. *et al.* (1996) Lack of effect of long term supplementation with beta carotene on the incidence of malignant neoplasms and cardiovascular disease. *N. Engl. J. Med.*, **334**: 1145–1149.

Hertog, M.G.L., Feskens, E.J.M., Hollman, P.C.H. *et al.* (1993) Dietary antioxidant flavonoids and risk of coronary heart disease: the Zutphen Elderly Study. *Lancet*, **342**: 1007–1011.

Hirai, A., Terano, T., Hamazaki, T. *et al.* (1982) The effects of the oral administration of fish oil concentrate on the release and the metabolism of [^{14}C] arachidonic acid and [^{14}C] eicosapentaenoic acid by human platelets. *Thromb. Res.*, **28**: 285–298.

Hjermann, I., Velve-Byre, K., Holme, I. and Leren, P. (1981) Effect of diet and smoking intervention on incidence of CHD: report from the Oslo study group of a randomised trial in healthy men. *Lancet*, **2**: 1303–1310.

Hodgson, J.M., Wahlqvist, M.L., Boxall, J.A. *et al.* (1993) Can linoleic acid contribute to coronary artery disease? *Am. J. Clin. Nutr.*, **58**: 228–234.

Holland, B., Welch, A., Unwin, I., Buss, D., Paul, A. and Southgate, D. (1991) *The Composition of Foods*, 5th edn, Royal Society of Chemistry, London.

Hopkins, P.N. (1992) Effects of dietary cholesterol on serum cholesterol: a meta-analysis and review. *Am. J. Clin. Nutr.*, **55**: 1060–1070.

Hseih, S.D. and Yoshinaga, H. (1995) Abdominal fat distribution and coronary heart disease risk factors in men – waist/height ratio as a simple and useful predictor. *Int. J. Obesity*, **19**: 585–589.

Intersalt Cooperative Research Group (1988)

Intersalt: an international study of electrolyte excretion and blood pressure. Results for 24 hour urinary sodium and potassium excretion. *Br. Med. J.*, **297**: 319–328.

Isles, C.G., Hole, D.J., Gillis, C.R., Hawthorne, V.M. and Lever, A.F. (1989) Plasma cholesterol, coronary heart disease and cancer in the Renfrew and Paisley survey. *Br. Med. J.*, **298**: 920–924.

Jacobs, D., Blackburn, H., Higgins, M. *et al.* (1992) Report of the Conference on low blood cholesterol: mortality associations. *Circulation*, **86**: 1046–1060.

Jenkins, D.J.A., Wolever, T.M.S. and Taylor, R.H. (1981) Dietary fibre, fibre analogues and glucose transport: importance of viscosity. *Am. J. Clin. Nutr.*, **34**: 362–366.

Jenkins, D.J.A. *et al.* (1989) Nibbling versus gorging: metabolic advantages of increased meal frequency. *N. Engl. J. Med.*, **321**: 929–934.

Jenkins, D.J.A., Wolever, T.M.S., Rao, A.V. *et al.* (1993) Effect on blood lipids of very high intakes of fiber in diets low in saturated fat and cholesterol. *N. Engl. J. Med.*, **329**: 21–26.

Kang, S., Wong, P.W.K., Susmano, A., Sora, J., Norusis, M. and Ruggie, N. (1991) Thermolabile methylenetetrahydrofolate reductase. *Am. J. Hum. Genet.*, **48**: 536–545.

Kannel, W.B. and Gordon, T. (eds) (1970) *Some characteristics related to the incidence of cardiovascular disease and death. The Framingham Study; 6 year follow up.* US Govt Printing Office, Washington, DC.

Kannel, W.B., Neaton, J.D., Wentworth, D. *et al.* (1986) Overall and coronary heart disease mortality rates in relation to major risk factors in 325,348 men screened for MRFIT. *Am. Heart J.*, **112**: 825–836.

Keys, A. (1957) Diet and the epidemiology of Coronary Heart Disease. *JAMA*, **164**: 1912–1919.

Keys, A. (1970) Coronary heart disease in seven countries. *Circulation*, **41**: 1–211.

Keys, A. (1980) *Seven Countries: A Multivariate Analysis of Death and Coronary Heart Disease*, Howard University Press, London.

Knekt, P., Jarvinen, R., Reunanen, A. *et al.* (1996) Flavonoid intake and coronary mortality in Finland: a cohort study. *Br. Med. J.*, **312**: 478–481.

Kushi, L.H., Folsom, A.R., Prineas, R.J. *et al.* (1996). Dietary antioxidant vitamins and death from coronary heart disease in postmenopausal women. *N. Engl. J. Med.*, **334**: 1156–1162.

Lapidus, L., Bengtsson, B., Larsson, B., Pennert, R., Rybo, E. and Bjostrom, L. (1984) Distribution of adipose tissue and risk of CVD and death: a 12 year follow up of participants in the population study of women in Gothenburg, Sweden. *Br. Med. J.*, **288**: 1257–1261.

Law, M.K., Frost, C.D. and Wald, N.J. (1991) By how much does dietary salt reduction lower blood pressure? *Br. Med. J.*, **302**: 811–819.

Law, M.R., Thompson, S.G. and Wald, N.J. (1994) Assessing possible hazards of reducing serum cholesterol. *Br. Med. J.*, **308**: 373–379.

Lawn, R.M. (1992) Lipoprotein(a) in heart disease. *Scientific American*, **June**: 26–32.

Lean, M.E.J., Han, T.S. and Morrison, C.E. (1995) Waist circumference as a measure for indicating need for weight management. *Br. Med. J.*, **311**: 158–161.

Lejeune, S.R.E., Ashwell, M.A., Cox, B.D. and Whichelow, M.J. Waist:height ratio is a simple anthropometric index which is closely associated with blood pressure in middle-aged adults. *Proc. Nutr. Soc* (in press).

Linn, S., Fulwood, R., Rifkind, B. *et al.* (1989) High density lipoprotein cholesterol levels among US adults by selected demographic and socioeconomic variables. *Am. J. Epidemiol.*, **129**: 281–294.

MacMahon, S., Peto, R., Culter, J. *et al.* (1990) Blood pressure, stroke and coronary heart disease. Part 1, Prolonged differences in blood pressure: prospective observational studies corrected for the regression dilution bias. *Lancet*, **335**: 765–774.

MAFF (1994a) *The Dietary and Nutritional Survey of British Adults – Further Analysis.* HMSO, London.

MAFF (1994b) *National Food Survey, 1993.*

MAFF (1995) *National Food Survey, 1994.*

MAFF, DH, HEA (1990) *Eight Guidelines for a Healthy Diet*, Food Sense, London.

Manson, J.E., Tosteson, H., Ridker, P.M. *et al.* (1992) The primary prevention of myocardial infarction. *N. Engl. J. Med.*, **326**: 1406–1416.

Manson, J.E., Willett, W.C., Stampfer, M.J. *et al.* (1995) Body weight and mortality among women. *N. Engl. J. Med.*, **333**: 677–685.

Markowe, H.L.J. (1985) Fibrinogen: a possible link between social class and coronary heart disease. *Br. Med. J.*, **291**: 1312–1314.

Marmot, M.G., Rose, G. and Shipley, M. (1978) Employment grade and CHD in British civil servants. *J. Epidemiol. Commun. Health*, **32**: 244–249.

McCully, K.S. (1969) Vascular pathology of homocysteinemia; implications for the pathogenesis of arteriosclerosis. *Am. J. Pathol.*, **56**: 111–128.

McGrath, S.A. and Gibney, M.J. (1994) The effects of altered frequency of eating on plasma lipids in free-living healthy males on normal self-selected diets. *Eur. J. Clin. Nutr.*, **48**: 402–407.

McKeigue, P.M., Marmot, M.G., Adelstein, A.M. *et*

al. (1985) Diet and risk factors for coronary heart disease in Asians in Northwest London. *Lancet*, **ii**: 1086–1090.

McKeigue, P.M., Shah, B. and Marmot, M.G. (1991) Relation of central obesity and insulin resistance with high diabetes prevalence and cardiovascular risk in South Asians. *Lancet*, **337**: 382–386.

McNamara, D.J. (1990) Relationship between blood and dietary cholesterol. In *Meat and Health. Advances in Meat Research* (eds A.M. Pearson and T.R. Dutson), London, pp. 63–87.

Meade, T.W., Mellows, S., Brozovic, M. *et al.* (1986) Haemostatic function and ischaemic heart disease : principal results of the Northwick Park Heart Study. *Lancet*, **2**: 533–537.

Meade, T.W., Ruddock, V., Stirling, Y. *et al.* (1993) Fibrinolytic activity, clotting factors, and long-term incidence of ischaemic heart disease in the Northwick Park Heart Study. *Lancet*, **342**: 1076–1079.

Mensink, R.P. and Katan, M.B. (1990) Effects of dietary trans fatty acids on high density and low density lipoprotein levels in healthy subjects. *N. Engl. J. Med.*, **323**: 439–444.

Miller, G.J., Stirling, Y., Howarth, D.J. *et al.* (1995) Dietary fat intake and plasma factor VII antigen concentration. *Thromb. Haemost.*, **73**: 893.

MRC Working Party (1988) Stroke and CHD in mild hypertension: risk factors and the value of treatment. *Br. Med. J.*, **296**: 1565–1572.

Muldoon, M.F., Manuc, S.B. and Matthews, J.A. (1990) Lowering cholesterol concentrations and mortality : a quantitative review of primary prevention trials. *Br. Med. J.*, **301**: 309–314.

National Research Council (1989) *Recommended daily allowances*, l0th edn. Food and Nutrition Board, Nut. Aca. Sci. USA, Washington, DC.

O'Flaherty, L. and Gibney, M.J. (1994) The effect of very low-, moderate- and high-fat snacks on postprandial reverse cholesterol transport in healthy volunteers. (abs.) *Proc. Nutr. Soc.* **53** 3: 124.

Oliver, M.F. (1995) Statins prevent coronary heart disease. *Lancet*, **346**: 1378–1379.

Omenn, G.S., Goodman, G.E., Thornquist, M.D. *et al.* (1996) Effects of a combination of beta carotene and vitamin A on lung cancer and cardiovascular disease. *N. Engl. J. Med.*. **334**: 1150–1155.

Paneth, N. and Susser, M. (1995) Early origins of coronary heart disease (the 'Barker hypothesis') *Br. Med. J.*, **310**: 411–412.

Patel, P., Mendall, M.A., Carrington, D. *et al.* (1995) Association of *Helicobacter pylori* and *Chlamydia* pneumoniae infections with coronary heart disease and cardiovascular risk factors. *Br. Med. J.*, **311**: 711–714.

Patsch, J.R. (1987) Postprandial lipaemia. *Baillère's Clin. Endocrinol. Metab.*, **1**: 551–571.

Pekkanen, J., Linn, S., Heiss, G. *et al.* (1990) Ten year mortality from cardiovascular disease in relation to cholesterol level among men with and without pre-existing cardiovascular disease. *N. Engl. J. Med.*, **322**: 1700–1707.

Perry, I.J., Refsum, H., Morris, R.W. *et al.* (1995) Prospective study of serum total homocysteine concentration and risk of stroke in middle aged British men. *Lancet*, **346**: 1395–1398.

Peto, R., Boreham, J., Chen, J. *et al.* (1989) Plasma cholesterol, coronary heart disease and cancer. *Br. Med. J.*, **298**: 1249.

Pocock, S.J., Shaper, A.G., Cook, D.G. *et al.* (1987) Social class differences in ischaemic heart disease in British men. *Lancet*, **2**: 197–201.

Pocock, S.J., Shaper, A.G. and Phillips, A.N. (1989) Concentrations of high density lipoprotein cholesterol, triglycerides and total cholesterol in ischaemic heart disease. *Br. Med. J.*, **298**: 998–1002.

Ramsay, L., Yeo, W. and Jackson, P. (1991) Dietary reduction of serum cholesterol concentrations: time to think again. *Br. Med. J.*, **303**: 953–957.

Ravnskov, U. (1992) Cholesterol lowering trials in coronary heart disease: frequency of citation and outcome. *Br. Med. J.*, **305**: 15-19.

Regenstrom, J., Nilsson, J., Tornvall, P., Landou, C. and Hausten, A. (1992) Susceptibility to low density lipoprotein oxidation and coronary atherosclerosis in man. *Lancet*, **339**: 1183–1186.

Renaud, S. and de Lorgeril, M. (1992) Wine, alcohol, platelets and the French paradox for coronary heart disease. *Lancet*, **339**: 1523–1526.

Renaud, S., Godsey, F., Dument, E., Thevenan, C., Ortchanian, E. and Martin, J.L. (1986) Influence of long-term diet modification on platelet function and composition in Moselle farmers. *Am. J. Clin. Nutr.*, **43**: 136–150.

Ridker, P.M., Hennekens, C.H. and Stampfer, M.J. (1993) A prospective study of lipoprotein(a) and the risk of myocardial infarction. *JAMA*, **270**: 2195–2199.

Riemersma, R.A., Oliver, M., Elton, R.A. *et al.* (1990) Plasma antioxidants and coronary heart disease: vitamins C and E, and selenium. *Eur. J. Clin. Nutr.*, **44**: 143-150.

Riemersma, R.A., Wood, D.A., Macintyre, C.C.A., Elton, R.A., Gey, K.F. and Oliver, M.F. (1991a) Antioxidants and pro-oxidants in coronary heart disease. *Lancet*, **337**: 667.

Riemersma, R.A., Wood, D.A., Macintyre, C.C.A., Elton, R.A., Gey, K.F. and Oliver, M.F. (1991b) Risk of angina pectoris and plasma concentrations of vitamins A, C and E and carotene. *Lancet*, **337**: 1–5.

Rimm, E.B., Stampfer, M.D., Ascherio, A., Giovannucci, M., Colditz, G.A. and Willett, W.C. (1993) Vitamin E consumption and the risk of coronary heart disease in men. *N. Engl. J. Med.*, **328**: 1450–1455.

Rimm, E.B., Klatskey, A., Grobbee, D. *et al.* (1996) Review of moderate alcohol consumption and reduced risk of coronary heart disease: is the effect due to beer, wine, or spirits? *Br. Med. J.*, **312**: 731–736.

Ripsin, C.M., Keenan, J.M., Jacobs, D.R. *et al.* (1992) Oat products and lipid lowering – a metaanalysis. *JAMA*, **267**: 3317–3325.

Sadler, M., Ashwell, M. and Arens, U. (1995) Food, heart disease and stroke (Conference summary). *BNF Nutr. Bull.*, **20**: 34–41.

Salonen, J.T., Salonen, R., Seppanen, K., Kantola, M., Suntioinen, S. and Korpela, H. (1991) Interactions of serum copper, selenium and low density lipoprotein cholesterol in atherogenesis. *Br. Med. J.*, **302**: 756–760.

Salonen, J.T., Yla-Herttuala, S., Yamamoto, R. *et al.* (1992a) Autoantibody against oxidised LDL and progression of carotid atherosclerosis. *Lancet*, **339**: 883–887.

Salonen, J.T., Nyyssonen, K., Korpelu, H., Tuomilehto, J., Seppanen, R. and Salonen, R. (1992b) High stored iron levels are associated with excess risk of myocardial infarction in Eastern Finnish men. *Circulation*, **86**: 803–811.

Sanchez-Castillo, C.P., Warrender, S., Whitehead, T.P. and James, W.P.T. (1987) An assessment of the sources of dietary salt in a British population. *Clin. Sci.*, **72**: 95–102.

Sanders, T.A.B. and Roshanai, F. (1984) Assessment of fatty acid intakes in vegans and omnivores. *Hum. Nutr. Appl. Nutr.*, **38A**: 345–354.

Selhub, J., Jacqes, P.F., Bostom, A.G. *et al.* (1995) Association between plasma homocysteine levels and extracranial carotid artery stenosis. *N. Engl. J. Med.*, **332**: 286–291.

Shaper, A.G. (1988) *Coronary Heart Disease: Risks and Reasons*, Current Medical Literature Ltd, London.

Shaper, A.G., Pocock, S.J., Walker, M., Cohen, N.M., Wale, C.J. and Thomson, A.G. (1981) British Regional Heart Study: cardiovascular risk factors in middle-aged men in 24 towns. *Br. Med. J.*, **283**: 179–186.

Shekelle, R.B., MacMillan Shryock, A., Paul, O., Lepper, M., Stamler, J., Liu, S. and Rayner, W.J. (1981) Diet, serum cholesterol and death from coronary heart disease. The Western Electric Study. *N. Engl. J. Med.*, **304**: 65–70.

Stampfer, M.J. and Malinow, M.R. (1995) Can lowering homocysteine levels reduce cardiovascular disease? *N. Engl. J. Med.*, **332**: 328–329.

Stampfer, M.J., Malinow, M.R., Willet, W.C. *et al.* (1992) A prospective study of plasma homocysteine and risk of myocardial infarction in US physicians. *JAMA*, **268**: 877–881.

Stampfer, M.J., Hennekens, C.H., Manson, J.E., Colditz, G.A., Rosner, B, and Willett, W.C. (1993) Vitamin E consumption and the risk of coronary disease in women. *N. Engl. J. Med.*, **328**: 1444–1449.

Steinberg, D., Parthasarthy, S., Carew, T.E. *et al.* (1989) Beyond cholesterol: modications of low-density lipoproteins that increase its atherogenicity. *N. Engl. J. Med.*, **320**: 915–924.

Stephens, N.G., Parsons, A., Schofield, P.M. *et al.* (1996) Randomised controlled trial of vitamin E in patients with coronary disease: Cambridge Heart Antioxidant Study (CHAOS). *Lancet*, **347**: 781–786.

Strachan, D.P., Leon, D.A. and Dodgeon, B. (1995) Mortality from cardiovascular disease among interregional migrants in England and Wales. *Br. Med. J.*, **310**: 423–427.

Swales, J. (1992) Salt and blood pressure. *Blood Press.*, **1**: 201–204.

The Alpha-Tocopherol, Beta Carotene Cancer Prevention Study Group (1994) The effect of vitamin E and beta carotene on the incidence of lung cancer and other cancers in male smokers. *N. Engl. J. Med.*, **330**: 1029–1081.

Turpeinen, U., Karvonen, M.J., Pekkarinea, M., Miettinen, M., Elosuo, K. and Paavilainen, E. (1979) Dietary prevention of coronary heart disease: the Finnish mental hospital study. *Int. J. Epidemiol.*, **8**: 99–118.

Ubbink, J.B. (1995) Homocysteine – an atherogenic and a thrombogenic factor? *Nutr. Rev.*, **53**: 323–325.

Ulbricht, T.L.V. and Southgate, D.A.T. (1991) Coronary heart disease: seven dietary factors. *Lancet*, **338**: 985–992.

van der Kooy, K. (1993) *Changes in body composition and fat distribution in response to weight loss and weight regain.* PhD Thesis, CIP-Gegevens Koninjluke Biobioltheek, The Hague.

Van Houwelingen, A.C., Hornstra, G., Krombout, D. and Coulander, C. (1989) Habitual fish consumption, fatty acids of serum phospholipids and platelet function. *Atherosclerosis*, **75**: 157–165.

Victor, R.G. and Hansen, J. (1995) Alcohol and blood pressure – a drink a day. *N. Engl. J. Med.*, **332**: 1782–1783.

Widdowson, E.M. (1974) Changes in pigs due to undernutrition before birth and for one, two and three years afterwards and the effects of rehabilitation. *Adv. Exp. Med. Biol.*, **49**: 165–181.

Willett, W.C., Stampfer, M.J., Manson, J.E. *et al.* (1993) Intake of trans fatty acids and risk of coronary heart disease among women. *Lancet*, **341**: 581–585.

Williams, C. (1995) Healthy eating: clarifying advice about fruit and vegetables. *Br. Med. J.*, **310**: 1453–1455.

Williams, C.M., Zampelas, A., Jackson, K.G. *et al.* (1995) Postprandial triacyglycerol responses to meals of varying monounsaturated fatty acid content in UK and Greek subjects. *Atherosclerosis*, **115**: 846.

Witzum, J.L. (1994) The oxidation hypothesis of atherosclerosis. *Lancet*, **344**: 793–795.

World Health Organization (1989) *World Statistics Annual.* WHO, Geneva.

World Health Organization (1990) *Diet, nutrition and the prevention of chronic diseases.* Report of a WHO Study Group. Technical Report Series no. 797, WHO, Geneva.

World Health Organization (1992) *World Statistics Annual.* WHO, Geneva.

Zampelas, A. (1994) Postprandial lipaemia, coronary heart disease and dietary fatty acid composition. In *Tomorrow's Nutrition 1994* (eds M. Ashwell and M. Sadler), Proceedings of the 16th British Nutrition Foundation Annual Conference, British Nutrition Foundation, London: 25–36.

Zavaroni, I., Bonoera, E., Pagliari, M. *et al.* (1989) Risk factors for coronary artery disease in healthy persons with hyperinsulinaemia and normal glucose tolerance. *N. Engl. J. Med.*, **320**: 702–706.

Zilversmit, A.B. (1979) Atherogenesis: a postprandial phenomenon. *Circulation*, **60**: 473–475.

GLOSSARY

Angina Chest pain indicating impaired blood supply to the heart muscle.

Antioxidant A compound which prevents or protects against the damage which could be caused by the oxidation of fatty acids and proteins by free radicals.

Apoprotein A protein which transports fat-soluble substances in the blood.

ApoproteinA (apoA) The additional apoprotein associated with lipoprotein(a).

ApoproteinB (apoB) The major protein of low density lipoprotein.

Arrhythmia Any form of irregular electrical activity in heart muscle leading to irregular heart beat. It can be intermittent or continuous.

Atherosclerosis The process leading to the thickening of artery walls by the deposition of cholesterol fatty acids and blood clots.

Blood pressure (BP) The pressure of blood in the main arteries. *Systolic* blood pressure is the high pressure and occurs when the heart is contracting. *Diastolic* blood pressure is the lowest pressure and occurs when the heart is relaxing.

Body mass index (BMI) Weight (kg)/height^2(m^2).

British Regional Heart Study An ongoing study begun in 1978 of 7735 men, 40 to 59 years in 24 towns in the UK, studying all major risk factors.

Cardiovascular disease (CVD) A broad term encompassing coronary heart disease, peripheral atherosclerosis and stroke.

Carotenoids Naturally occurring pigments found in vegetables and fruits that have antioxidant activity. β-carotene is the main source of dietary provitamin A. It has a structure identical with vitamin A in both halves of the molecule. Most of the other carotenoids e.g. xanthophyll and lycopene have no provitamin A activity.

Central fat distribution The pattern of fat distribution in the body where fat stores are mainly deposited internally in the trunk and abdomen.

***cis* Fatty acids** Monounsaturated fatty acids with a double bond in which the position of the hydrogen atoms causes a pronounced kink in the chain. Lipids containing *cis*-fatty acids cannot pack so closely together. They are commonly found in natural lipids.

Coagulation cascade The series of reactions which produces a fibrin network.

Dietary and Nutritional Survey of British Adults A survey of the dietary behaviour, nutritional status and blood pressure of about 2000 UK adults aged 16 to 64 years, carried out in 1986–1987.

Dietary reference values (DRVs) A term covering estimates for nutrient requirements.

Docosahexaenoic acid (DHA) A fatty acid of the n-3 series with 22 carbon atoms and 6 double bonds.

Eicosanoids Highly active derivatives of the 20 carbon fatty acids, di-homo-gamma linolenic acid, arachidonic acid (20:4 n-6) and eicosapentaenoic acid, such as prostacyclin and thromboxanes, that have varied and frequently opposing physiological effects.

Eicosapentaenoic acid (EPA) A fatty acid of the n-3 series with 20 carbon atoms and 5 double bonds.

Endothelial cells A single layer of cells lining the inside of the artery.

Essential fatty acids (EFA) Fatty acids (linoleic acid and α-linolenic acid) that are not made in the body and must be supplied in the diet.

Factor VII A clotting factor in the blood.

Familial hypercholesterolaemia An inherited tendency towards extremely high plasma cholesterol levels often resulting in premature CHD death.

Fibrinogen/fibrin Fibrinogen is converted into fibrin at the end of the coagulation cascade producing a network of fibrin strands.

Fibrinolysis The process by which a blood clot is dissolved.

Fibrous plaque The fatty fibrous lesion on the artery wall.

Foam cells One of the early signs of atherosclerosis; large cells in the artery wall full of fatty acids and cholesterol.

Framingham Study An ongoing study begun in the 1940s of about 5000 men and women, studying all major risk factors for CHD.

Free radicals Highly active oxygen-derived species (radicals) (e.g. hydroxyl and superoxide) which have the capacity to damage cellular components by oxidation.

Glycaemic Index (GI) Relative rates of glucose absorption from different foods.
HDL-cholesterol High density lipoprotein cholesterol; the form in which cholesterol is removed from the tissues and returned to the liver.
Hyperlipidaemia Raised levels of blood lipids.
INTERSALT An international epidemiological study in 52 centres measuring blood pressure, urinary sodium excretion, body mass index and alcohol intake.
Intima The second innermost layer of the artery wall.
Insulin The hormone which causes glucose to be removed from the blood and taken up by the tissues when glucose levels are high.
Insulin resistance A condition in which cells are resistant to the action of insulin and more is required to achieve the same effect.
Lipoprotein The form in which lipids are transported in the blood.
Lipoprotein(a) (Lp(a)) A lipoprotein similar to low density lipoprotein, but with an additional apoprotein – apoproteinA.
LDL-cholesterol Low density lipoprotein cholesterol; the form in which cholesterol is transported from the liver to the tissues.
Lumen The space within the artery, through which the blood flows.
Macrophage Large cells which remove bacteria and other foreign particles from the blood.
Media The middle layer in the artery wall. It is composed of smooth muscle cells which control the diameter of the artery.
Meta-analysis Overall analysis of data from a number of large studies or trials.
Multiple Risk Factor Intervention Trial (MRFIT) An intervention study carried out in the 1970s involving 13 000 men, aged 35 to 37 years. The experimental group were given advice about diet, smoking and high blood pressure.
Myocardial infarction The lack of blood and oxygen supply to an area of heart muscle due to blockage in the coronary arteries. In severe cases, it can cause the heart to stop beating and is fatal.
Non-starch polysaccharides (NSP) The major fraction of dietary fibre that is chemically identifiable and can be measured with reasonable precision.
Oxidized-LDL Low density lipoprotein that is altered chemically by oxidation of its constituent polyunsaturated fatty acids. This alters the apoprotein so that it is not recognized by normal receptors.
P/S ratio The ratio of polyunsaturated to saturated fatty acids in the diet.
Peripheral fat distribution The pattern of fat distribution around the body where fat is mainly deposited subcutaneously around the thighs and hips.
Platelet Small blood cells which are involved in blood clotting.
Platelet aggregation The process by which platelets are induced to clump together and form larger aggregates. These become enmeshed in the fibrin network.
Pro-oxidants Substances promoting oxidation.
Propionate A short-chain fatty acid produced by colonic bacteria from fermentation of non-starch polysaccharides and resistant starch.
Prostacyclin(s) Powerful vasodilators and inhibitors of platelet aggregation that are released from endothelial cells.
Resistant starch Starch that is not digested by enzymes in the small intestine and passes into the colon where it is fermented by the colonic bacteria.
Risk factor A factor associated with the onset and progression of disease.
Scavenger receptor Receptors on macrophages which recognize the oxidized forms of LDL-cholesterol.
Seven Countries Study Data was obtained during 1957–1962 with follow-up 5–10 years later, on all major risk factors, but particularly saturated fat intake and blood cholesterol levels, for a total of 12 000 men, 40 to 59 years, across seven countries – Japan, Greece, Italy, Finland, USA, former Yugoslavia and Holland.
Short-chain fatty acids The type of fatty acids produced by colonic bacteria from fermentation of non-starch polysaccharides and resistant starch.
Soluble non-starch polysaccharides Pectic substances and plant gums that are soluble in water.
Syndrome X A pattern of metabolic disorders resulting in a clustering of risk factors, termed the insulin resistance syndrome that is strongly associated with central fat distribution.
Thrombogenesis Formation of a thrombus.
Thrombosis The condition in which a blood clot blocks an artery and stops the blood flow through it.
Thrombus A blood clot formed in a blood vessel.
Thromboxane(s) Produced by platelets and stimulate platelet aggregation and vasoconstriction.
***trans* Fatty acids** Fatty acids with double bonds that adopt a configuration allowing the chains to pack closely together. They are mainly produced during hydrogenation of vegetables, although a few occur naturally.
Triglyceride A fat consisting of three fatty acids on a glycerol backbone.
Unit of alcohol 8 g or 10 ml of ethyl alcohol.
Whitehall Civil Servants Study During 1967 and 1969 data were collected for all major risk factors, particularly employment status, on 17 530 male civil servants in London.
WHO World Health Organization

INDEX

Page numbers appearing in **bold** refer to figures; page numbers appearing in *italic* refer to tables.

The BNF is an impartial scientific organization which sets out to provide reliable information and scientifically based advice on nutrition and related health matters, with the ultimate objective of helping individuals to understand how they may best match their diet with their lifestyle. Its principal functions fall under the headings of information, education and research.

The BNF is a non-profit making organization, registered as a charity. Its work is principally funded by donations from its membership. The Foundation draws upon the expert knowledge and extensive experience of the eminent members of its Council and committees. Their support underpins and underwrites the Foundation's integrity and reputation.

MIX
Papier aus verantwortungsvollen Quellen
Paper from responsible sources
FSC® C105338

If you have any concerns about our products,
you can contact us on
ProductSafety@springernature.com

In case Publisher is established outside the EU,
the EU authorized representative is:
Springer Nature Customer Service Center GmbH
Europaplatz 3, 69115 Heidelberg, Germany

Printed by Libri Plureos GmbH
in Hamburg, Germany